God, Faith, and Health

Exploring the Spirituality-Healing Connection

Jeff Levin, Ph.D.

John Wiley & Sons, Inc.

New York • Chichester • Weinheim • Brisbane • Singapore • Toronto

Library of Congress Cataloging-in-Publication Data

Levin, Jeffrey S.
    God, faith, and health : exploring the spirituality-health connection
/ Jeff Levin.
        p.   cm.
Includes bibliographical references.
    ISBN 0-471-35503-8 (cloth : alk. paper)
    1.   Health–Religious aspects.   I. Title.
    BL65.M4 L48 2001
    291.1'78321–dc21   2001017861

To Lea, my precious one.

Contents

Foreword

Future historians of medicine will describe the twentieth century as the period in which spirituality, after a long absence, began to return to healing, and they will mark Jeff Levin as one of the greatest architects of this development. It is rare that someone establishes a completely new field in medicine, but that is what Dr. Levin has done. His scholarship has led to the emergence of what he calls "the epidemiology of religion," which focuses on the relationship of religious practices to health.

Most people outside of medicine take for granted the idea that religious practices such as worship, prayer, and meditation are important for their health, and they often wonder what the fuss over these issues is all about. But the fact is, unfortunately, that medical science has long looked with disdain on the possibility of a spiritual factor in health. For most of the twentieth century, we physicians have insisted that health is determined solely by what the atoms and molecules in the body happen to be doing, which is following the so-called blind laws of nature. Generations of physicians have viewed with skepticism and often with ridicule the possibility that our patients' religious views and spiritual practices might make a difference in their health. But today our patients are having the last laugh. As Levin compellingly shows, people who follow a religious path are more likely to enjoy greater longevity and a higher quality of health than those who do not. To be sure, there is no *guarantee* of such a benefit for any given individual, as Levin is careful to state. As with all therapies doctors employ, these results are statistical in nature and are based on averages.

Levin's findings have created immense interest in the medical profession because they rest on a powerful word: *data*. Almost no one knew that this evidence existed before Levin unearthed it and brought it to the attention of physicians. The reason it remained hidden was that we were blind to it, in spite of the fact that it was in plain sight. Why was it so difficult to see?

As medicine became increasingly mechanical from the mid-nineteenth century onward, most people believed that the future of health care lay almost totally in a technical direction. As the break-throughs steadily appeared—anesthesia, vaccines, antibiotics, surgical advances, and most recently, genetic manipulation—physicians often felt that the victory celebration over disease might break out at any moment. Against this backdrop, the evidence of a role for spiritual factors in health was obscured. When it emerged through Levin's work, it was totally unanticipated and caught many by surprise. But as this evidence has become widely known, medicine has steadily warmed to it. One of the best indicators of its acceptance is that currently between one-third and one-half of the medical schools in the United States have adopted courses exploring religious and spiritual factors in health.

When a factor is discovered that positively affects the health and longevity of human beings, it automatically becomes the responsibility of physicians to engage it and learn to use it for the benefit of their patients. Failing to do so would be irresponsible, like turning away from a new antibiotic or a new surgical procedure. That is why Levin's work is winning converts in medical schools, hospitals, and clinics throughout the world.

Even so, there are, predictably, a few cynics who decry these developments. Some doggedly insist, ostrichlike, that the evidence Levin demonstrates does not exist. They insist that religion and science do not mix, and that attempts to bring them together are, as one skeptic put it, "horrendous and evil." They see Levin's efforts as an attempt to steer medicine back to the Dark Ages. They take the dour view that emphasizing spiritual factors in health will only make people feel guilty when they get sick; that religion is too delicate and personal for physicians to explore; and that these matters should therefore be left to ministers and priests. There is a grain of truth in these concerns—all therapies have side effects and can be abused—but they appear increasingly hollow when put to the test in hospitals, clinics, and physicians' offices across the land. Studies continue to show that the benefits of applying these findings far outweigh the potential problems involved. Many who object to Levin's findings seem to do so because of deeply held suspicions and prejudices against religion, which was illustrated in the comment of one skeptic who said, "This is the sort of thing I wouldn't believe, even if it were true."

Are these issues too personal for health care professionals to become involved in? The lessons of the past can help allay such worries. Not too long ago, physicians believed they should not inquire about the sexual practices and drinking habits of their patients. But as evidence mounted that these were important health issues, physicians began to inquire about them with the appropriate sensitivity. Today it would be considered malpractice to avoid these areas. In the same way, physicians can learn to interact skillfully and gently regarding their patients' spiritual life, to the benefit of their health.

Perhaps the major challenge we face is how to avoid trivializing religious and spiritual practices. When laypersons and professionals discover the impact of these measures on health, they may begin to regard them as the latest item in the medical tool kit. Seen in this way, prayer becomes merely the latest aspirin, the newest penicillin. Prayer and spiritual practices have far greater benefits, I believe, than aiding physical health. They are our bridge to the Absolute, however named—God, Goddess, Allah, Universe, Tao. In my view, this benefit of religion dwarfs any physical advantage it may convey.

Levin's contributions just might lead to a respiritualization not just of medicine but of science in general. The idea that science can be conducted as a sacred, holy pursuit is foreign to most scientists; but in the early days of experimental science, a different view existed. The British chemist Robert Boyle, for example, the author of Boyle's Law, called scientists "priests of nature." He believed experiments were so sacred that they should be performed on Sundays, as part of the scientist's Sabbath worship.

This book should come with a warning: it can be a shock to anyone confronting this field for the first time. I shall never forget my own surprise when I first stumbled across a scientific study of intercessory prayer in hospitalized patients with heart attacks. It never occurred to me that religious practices such as prayer could be assessed like a new drug. At the time, I did not pray for my patients, and soon I found myself facing an ethical and moral dilemma. If this study was reliable, how could I justify *not* praying for my patients?

Withholding prayer might be the equivalent of denying them a valuable therapy, such as an antibiotic or surgical procedure. Did additional evidence exist? I embarked on a survey of all the scientific studies surrounding prayer and "distant healing" I could find. I was shocked to discover more than 130 experiments, not just in humans but also involving human tissue, animals, plants, and microorganisms. It was through this search that I discovered Jeff Levin's contributions, which impressed me tremendously because of their precision and far-reaching implications. I eventually came to regard these findings as one of the best-kept secrets in modern medicine. I began to incorporate private prayer in my practice of internal medicine, as an increasing number of physicians are also beginning to do.

No one should worry that religious practices and prayer are going to displace penicillin and surgery from medical care. Several national surveys have shown that Americans are extremely pragmatic when they get sick. They almost always use prayer *and* penicillin, not one or the other. When ill, "instead of" seems to be missing from their vocabulary. Americans want to cover *all* their bases. Therefore the skeptics' complaint that Levin's work will lure people away from using "real" medicine is almost totally without merit.

Levin is not selling religion or pushing any particular spiritual point of view. He does not dictate how anyone, including physicians, should respond to the information that follows. But it is clear that *some* response is necessary, and that this information should not be ignored. What should the response be? Should physicians inquire about their patients' religious beliefs and practices? Should doctors pray for those they serve? Levin wisely defers to physicians themselves on these questions. Some physicians may want to become personally involved. Others may feel more comfortable in suggesting that patients seek counsel from professionals such as ministers, priests, rabbis, pastoral counselors, or hospital chaplains.

The influence of religious and spiritual factors in health reflects a larger issue: the role of meaning in life. Without positive meaning, human life withers and health fails. For example, people who find nothing meaningful in their jobs have a higher rate of heart attack than do people who love their work. If the meaning of an occupation exerts life-and-death influences, it should not be surprising that spiritual meaning is also influential. Exploring how spiritual meaning affects health is the essence of this book.

When Sir Isaac Newton proposed the existence of universal gravity in the seventeenth century, it was considered such a radical idea that many of his colleagues condemned him as selling out to mysticism. But Newton stuck to his guns—data, evidence, experiments—and universal gravity was eventually vindicated and accepted. The same process is taking place today regarding the role of religion and spirituality in health. Some consider the idea fantastic, but the evidence says otherwise. As the supporting data continue to mount, it will not be long before physicians everywhere will be saying, "This is obvious!" And, as always happens when a new idea in science finally becomes accepted, there are those who will proclaim, "I thought of it first!"

In closing, I wish to express my personal gratitude to Dr. Jeff Levin for helping physicians rediscover what healers have known for more than 99.99 percent of the history of the human race: that spirituality is vital in health.

We need this lesson now more than ever.

Larry Dossey, M.D.
Author, *Reinventing Medicine*

Acknowledgments

God, Faith, and Health never would have been published without the enthusiastic support of my literary agent, Sandra Martin. I am indebted to Sandra for her determined efforts to find my book a home, and for her kind words of encouragement. Finding her was a godsend, which I also owe to our mutual friend, Gillian Spencer. I am also grateful to my editor, Tom Miller, and associate managing editor, Kimberly Monroe, for their patience as I wrote, and rewrote, this material, and for their considerable help in transforming my scientific jargon into readable prose.

Dr. Larry Dossey deserves some of the credit—and blame—for my decision to quit a successful career in academic medical research and pursue life as a writer and gentleman scientist. Larry had been pushing me for many years to write a book based on my research, and I am glad that I finally had the wisdom to listen. He has been a great friend and supporter, and sounding board, and he has my absolute respect as a visionary thinker without peer. Many of the wonderful things that have happened to me over the past decade have been due in part to the good words put in for me here and there by Larry.

Dr. David B. Larson also has been a supporter and valued colleague. When I left the academic world, Dave provided a "virtual" professional affiliation for me. The National Institute for Healthcare Research, a Rockville, Maryland, think tank that he founded, has administered my research and provided me with a title—senior research fellow—that I must admit sounds way cooler to me than associate professor.

The National Institutes of Health funded much of the research described in this book, both my own and that of many of the other scientists whose work is discussed. I am especially grateful to Dr. Katrina W. Johnson, who oversaw my early grant projects for the National Institute on Aging. Without Katrina's support, none of this work would have been funded. She pushed for acceptance of religious research within the NIH when it would have been politically more expedient not to do so. She is truly one of the unsung heroes of this whole field.

Dr. Robert Joseph Taylor and Dr. Linda M. Chatters, and more recently Dr. Christopher G. Ellison, have become wonderful friends and colleagues over the years. Our collaboration has been a highlight of my research career. Many of our studies, done alone or together, in various combinations, are described in the chapters to come. Robert, Linda, Chris, and I make a great team, and I hope that we will always find a way to work together in the future.

As a student many years ago, I began my work in this field in collaboration with three outstanding scientists and scholars: Drs. Preston L. Schiller, Kyriakos S. Markides, and Harold Y. Vanderpool. Their insights, in equal portion to my own, helped to shape my approach to the epidemiology of religion, and thus led directly to *God, Faith, and Health*. Harold and I cowrote a review essay in which we developed an explanatory framework for this field. That framework became the outline for this book.

My family was a great support to me as I wrote *God, Faith, and Health*. My mom and stepdad, Judith Citrin and Tom Wallace, and my dad and stepmom, Phil Citrin and Nanci Reichman, wondered at times if I had lost my mind in giving up a prestigious academic appointment, selling a dream house in Virginia Beach, giving away most of my possessions, and moving to Kansas to buy a farm and become a writer. Well, the verdict is still out on my sanity, but I hope that they can see my enhanced peace of mind...and I hope that they enjoy this book.

My grandpa, Harvey Goldfeder, of blessed memory, was a constant inspiration as I wrote this book. His remarkable life, nearly a century long, was a testament to the connection between spirituality and health. His confidence in me was unwavering, and I hope that I have honored him through my work.

I have been touched by the work of many great twentieth-century spiritual teachers of East and West, whose words and deeds have inspired me as I have tried to sort out the connections among body, mind, and spirit: Ram Dass, Paramahansa Yogananda, Meher Baba; and from my own tradition, Rabbi Zalman Schachter-Shalomi,

Rabbi Menachem Mendel Schneerson (*z"l*), Rabbi David A. Cooper, Rabbi Abraham Twerski, Rabbi Aryeh Kaplan (*z"l*), Rabbi Adin Steinsaltz, and especially Rabbi David Wolfe-Blank (*z"l*), whose creative genius enlightened my Torah learning each *Shabbat* for several years. I am grateful for their wisdom and insight.

Finally, I must give thanks and praise to the Lord God, Creator of All, for blessing me with my beloved Lea—a wife and partner whose love is my *yesod* and my *keter*, my foundation and my crown. "Grace is deceitful, and beauty is vain: but a woman who fears the Lord, she shall be praised." (Proverbs 31:30)

Jeff Levin

Introduction

Dr. Berton H. Kaplan stood at the front of the classroom, syllabus in hand. Thirty pairs of eyes eagerly awaited his instructions on the following week's assignment. After three hours of discussion, we were all tired and ready to go home. But Dr. Kaplan was a popular and respected teacher, so despite our weariness we were ready to receive our marching orders. More than twenty articles and chapters were assigned. I gulped hard, but did not complain. Even though the amount of reading was overwhelming—and I had four other classes—this was my favorite course and I had no doubt I would complete the assignment.

It was February 1982, and I was a first-year graduate student in the School of Public Health at the University of North Carolina in Chapel Hill. The course, "Culture and Health," was an advanced offering of the Department of Epidemiology. I could have signed up for a class with a lighter workload, but I knew I would enjoy learning about how thoughts, emotions, personality, and social relationships influenced patterns of health and illness.

Among the assigned readings were two articles on a most unusual topic. One had the intriguing if innocuous title "Frequency of Church Attendance and Blood Pressure Elevation." Findings were from a well-known study of adult men conducted by Dr. Thomas W. Graham and colleagues in Evans County, Georgia. For some reason, among the hundreds of questions asked of the study's participants was one on how often they attended church services. The authors had made a startling discovery: "A consistent pattern of lower systolic and diastolic blood pressures among frequent church attenders was found compared to that of infrequent attenders which was not due to the effects of age, obesity, cigarette smoking, or socioeconomic status."

In other words, men who attended church services at least once a week had significantly less hypertension than men who attended church less often. This finding was not due to the fact that the more religious men were less likely to smoke, or due to religious differences in other factors known to affect blood pressure, such as age, weight, or occupation. How could this be? Did going to church somehow prevent high blood pressure?

Fascinated, I read the next article, which was by Dr. Kaplan. In this thoughtful paper, "A Note on Religious Beliefs and Coronary Heart Disease," Dr. Kaplan reviewed several studies that found religious differences in rates of arteriosclerosis, heart attacks, deaths due to coronary artery disease, and other cardiovascular outcomes. Apparently, the Evans County study was not the only one on this topic.

Dr. Kaplan's essay closed with a statement that, though written in the dry academic style of medical journals, electrified me: "So we are left with a challenge to refine our concepts, and perfect our methodologies to see if, in fact, specific religious processes are related to the etiology, precipitation, recovery, or prevention of heart disease."

Little did I know that this sentence would set the stage for the next almost twenty years of my life, directing me to my life's work—the study of the connections between religious faith and health.

Medical Science Discovers Religion

The appearance over the past few years of cover stories in *Time*, *Reader's Digest*, and *Macleans*, articles in *Newsweek* and *USA Today*, and feature stories on shows as diverse as National Public Radio's "All Things Considered" and the Christian Broadcasting Network's "The 700 Club" attest to the public's interest in the possibility of a religion-health connection. Moreover, public interest seems to be growing. Just in the past couple years, stories have appeared on CBS, NBC, ABC, and NPR, and even in the *New York Times*.

Scientists, too, are becoming excited. Fascinating results are appearing regularly from researchers at such leading universities as Michigan, Yale, Duke, Berkeley, Rutgers, and Texas. Some findings are especially intriguing:

- People who regularly attend religious services have lower rates of illness and death than do infrequent or nonattenders.
- For each of the three leading causes of death in the United States—heart disease, cancer, and hypertension—people who report a religious affiliation have lower rates of illness.
- Older adults who participate in private and congregational religious activities have fewer symptoms, less disability, and lower rates of depression, chronic anxiety, and dementia.
- Religious participation is the strongest determinant of psychological well-being in African Americans—even more important than health or financial wealth.
- Actively religious people live longer, on average, than the nonreligious. This holds true even controlling for the fact that religious folks tend to avoid such behaviors as smoking and drinking that increase the risk of disease and death.

Remarkable findings like these are becoming commonplace in medical journals. Scientists have begun using the phrase "epidemiology of religion" to refer to this growing field of medical research. But just several years ago, few physicians and scientists knew that such data existed. Now, thanks to these studies, researchers have begun to realize that expressions of spirituality have measurable effects on health and well-being. This information is causing a revolution in medical research, medical education, and clinical practice.

Since 1990, the venerable National Institutes of Health (NIH), the federal agency responsible for supporting medical research throughout the United States, has funded studies of the health effects of religious involvement and spirituality. In 1995, NIH sponsored a conference for experts on technical issues in conducting scientific research in this area, and a separate conference for physicians and pastoral care professionals on assessing the spiritual domain. In 1996, NIH convened a special working group of academic scientists charged with developing more reliable and valid spiritual measures. Researchers and clinicians are now calling the NIH on a daily basis requesting information on this topic.

In 1996, the National Institute for Healthcare Research (NIHR), a private, not-for-profit think tank based in Rockville, Maryland, created a program to assist U.S. medical schools that wish to provide instruction on religion and spirituality to students and residents. Through NIHR's efforts, formal courses have been established at dozens of medical schools. In all, over half of U.S. medical schools now address spiritual topics in their curricula.

In 1997, even *JAMA*, the conservative journal of the American Medical Association (AMA), had to acknowledge that maybe, just maybe, there was something to this religion-health groundswell. In its September 3 issue, it published an article with the title "Religion and Spirituality in Medicine: Research and Education." The authors reviewed many of the same developments that will be described in this book, and urged physicians and medical educators to "become more aware of the importance of spirituality in patients' lives." The AMA is the staunch defender of orthodoxy in medicine. For them to publish—actually solicit—a paper with the words "religion" and "spirituality" in the title signals that this new field has received something of an official seal of approval by the medical establishment.

This rise to respectability for the religion-health connection has been especially gratifying for me. Beginning with the curiosity sparked in that classroom in 1982, it has been my good fortune to play a leading role in bringing the study of religion, spirituality, and health closer to the forefront. Most of the studies highlighted above were conducted by me and my collaborators. I wrote the earliest scholarly reviews of this field, received the first NIH grant, was an invited participant and keynote speaker at the two NIH conferences, and served on the NIH working group on religion and spirituality. A colleague and I coined the phrase "epidemiology of religion" for this field, and I was senior author of the article in *JAMA*. And it all began with a graduate school assignment nearly twenty years ago.

Spirituality: The Invisible Factor in Health

After that class session back in 1982, I could not get the Graham and Kaplan papers out of my mind. Each student was required to choose a topic for a term paper to be presented to the class, and I had found mine. With Dr. Kaplan's green light, I retreated to the health sciences library.

By the last week of class, I was done. When my turn came, I stood up in front of my classmates and spoke on "Religion as an Independent Variable in Epidemiology." I discussed in great detail the fifteen articles I had found in the library, most reporting statistical results from surveys or clinical investigations. Dr. Kaplan was very excited. He encouraged me to write up my findings for submission to a medical journal. Those few words were all I needed to set out on an adventure that would consume my nights and weekends for most of the next five years. Once again, I disappeared into the library. This time, though, I would not come up for air until 1987.

In those years, I began studies for my Ph.D. in preventive medicine and community health at the University of Texas Medical Branch in Galveston. Nearly every day after class, I burrowed through the stacks of the medical school library and immersed myself in the results of searches of the National Library of Medicine's *Index Medicus* and MEDLINE, a computerized database system. It quickly became clear that my initial count of fifteen published papers on religion and health was off—*way* off.

Along with the scores of biological, behavioral, and sociodemographic questions typically asked in health surveys, a stray religious question or two had managed to make a "guest appearance" in numerous studies in the past century. More often than not, a question on religion was included in the huge data-gathering expeditions typical of big studies; but with dozens of other results to report, researchers found little reason to give significant religious findings more than a brief mention. To most scientists and physicians, such findings were as good as invisible—no one seemed to be aware they existed.

As I located each of these studies, its details and findings were archived on a four-by-six index card. One afternoon, after placing an interlibrary loan request for an abstract published in an obscure Dutch subspecialty journal, I took a deep breath and decided to call it quits. Four and a half years after beginning my search, I pulled out all of my index cards and starting counting: I had found over *two hundred* studies! More than two hundred peer-reviewed articles reporting statistical findings on the impact of religious involvement on health and illness! I felt like a nineteenth-century explorer or archaeologist who had discovered something that no one else knew existed. I still have all of the articles and the box of yellowed index cards. I have not had the heart to throw them away.

In 1987, I published an article summarizing these results. This paper—"Is There a Religious Factor in Health?"—revealed that religious affiliation and involvement were clearly associated with patterns of health, disease, and death. To many people's amazement—and my own—it was clear that medical researchers had not just dabbled in religion. They had created a whole field, yet no one seemed to know that it was there. Despite claims to the contrary, which I still hear ("no one's ever looked at that"), there is scarcely a disease that has *not* been studied in relation to religion. Moreover, findings are remarkably consistent. They identify significant religious or spiritual effects on rates of health and illness regardless of the age, sex, race, ethnicity, nationality, or religious denomination of the people studied, and independent of the study design used and of when or where these studies took place. These findings have been confirmed and expanded on by contemporary studies conducted by scientists like me who are aware of this prior work and have investigated the health effects of religion and spirituality more directly and systematically.

How Medical Researchers Study
Religion and Spirituality

Before going further, it is important to say a few words about the field of *epidemiology*, the study of factors that promote health and prevent illness. This will help in understanding the research findings described throughout this book. Interpreting such data may seem tricky at first, but it is easy if a few simple principles are kept in mind.

Epidemiology uses scientific methods to describe patterns of health, disease, or death in a population by characteristics of person, place, or time. Studies that show different rates of breast cancer in different age groups, in different countries, or from year to year are examples of epidemiologic research. This approach is also used to investigate the impact of risk factors (such as tobacco smoking) or protective factors (such as exercise) on particular illnesses. Most research findings mentioned in the newspaper or on television every week—how some terrible new disease is on the rise or how a new factor has been shown to prevent a certain illness—are from epidemiologic studies.

Epidemiologists do something considered taboo in polite company: we make sweeping generalizations. An important thing to keep in mind when interpreting epidemiologic results is that findings are generally expressed (1) on average, (2) across a population, and (3) all things being equal. Epidemiology cannot tell us whether cigarettes caused Uncle Fred's emphysema—that requires the judgment of his physician. Epidemiology also cannot tell us whether quitting smoking might cure Fred's emphysema—that, too, requires the judgment of his physician, as well as analysis of the results of clinical research trials or intervention studies. But epidemiology can and does tell us that considerably more people who smoke cigarettes will develop emphysema and other awful diseases, and will die prematurely, compared to people who do not smoke. Likewise, a large body of research shows that folks who are religiously or spiritually involved, compared to those who are not, have a lower incidence of many diseases and a significantly lower death rate.

Does this mean that religious or spiritual people do not get sick? Of course not. Religious people certainly get sick and die, and many nonreligious people live long and healthy lives. But *on average*, it does appear that religious and spiritual involvement are associated with lower rates of illness and higher levels of well-being. In the language of epidemiology, this means that an active religious or spiritual life is a protective factor—much as a healthy diet and regular exercise are known protective factors. Still, many people who eat well and exercise regularly die suddenly at an early age, and many so-called couch potatoes who smoke, drink, and eat poorly live long and prosper.

This is an important point. Misinterpretation of research findings on religion, spirituality, and health may lead to confusion and unrealistic expectations as to the potential benefits of a spiritual way of life. Average findings produced by epidemiologists tend to hide or obscure the exceptions, such as people whose emotional well-being is harmed by religion. Further, the illness, suffering, or death of a particular person in no way should be—or can be—attributed to a lack of faith or not enough spirituality. Epidemiology is incapable of addressing such issues. What it can tell us—and does, very clearly—is that religious involvement deserves to be recognized as one of the significant factors that promote health and well-being among many groups of people.

Despite the volume of research findings supporting a religion-health connection, the concept remains controversial. Many scientists and physicians still dismiss it outright. Others who are more sympathetic but unaware of existing studies often state that there are no grounds for sound conclusions one way or the other. They are wrong. The evidence for a religious factor in health is, to quote another expert in this field, "overwhelming."

Dr. David B. Larson, physician and epidemiologist, is president of NIHR, the beltway think tank mentioned earlier. Prior to founding NIHR, Dr. Larson was on the faculty of Duke University Medical Center, a senior scientist and policymaker at the NIH, and a career commissioned officer in the U.S. Public Health Service. His résumé boasts more than two hundred scientific publications. Like me, Dr. Larson has devoted many years to reviewing the scientific evidence of a religion-health connection. He knows what the score is when it comes to the epidemiology of religion. And he is blunt: "While medical professionals have been privately assuming and publicly stating for years that religion is detrimental to mental health, when I actually looked at the available empirical research on the relationship between religion and health, the findings were overwhelmingly positive."

Just how positive is the subject of this book. The tacitly held view of scientists and physicians that "no one's ever looked at that" contrasts vividly with the sheer volume of research published over the past century. The idea that this is a forbidden or marginal topic for medical research no longer holds. Judging by the scientists publishing on this topic, the journals in which they publish, and the quality of the studies, the epidemiology of religion is clearly now in the mainstream of research on health and illness.

Religion versus Spirituality

A couple of terms appear throughout this book—terms that are often confused or used interchangeably. Historically, "religion" has denoted three things: particular churches or organized religious institutions (e.g., the Christian religion); a scholarly field of study; and the domain of life that deals with things of the spirit and matters of "ultimate concern." To talk of practicing religion or being religious refers to behaviors, attitudes, beliefs, experiences, and so on, that involve this domain of life. This is so whether one takes part in organized activities of an established religious institution or one has an inner life of the spirit apart from organized religions.

"Spirituality," as the term traditionally has been used, refers to a state of being that is acquired through religious devotion, piety, and observance. Attaining spirituality—union or connection with God or the divine—is an ultimate goal of religion, and is a state not everyone reaches. According to this usage, spirituality is a subset of a larger phenomenon, religion, and by definition is sought through religious participation. Religious scholars, historians, clergy and mystics of all faiths, and laypeople have always used the term in this way, almost without exception.

In the past twenty years or so, the word "spirituality" has taken on a new meaning. Popular writing by New Age authors and the media, often hostile to established religious institutions but open to private religious expression, have begun reserving the term "religion" for those behaviors, beliefs, and so forth that occur in the context of organized religion. All other religious expression, including practices like meditation and secular transcendent experiences (e.g., feelings of oneness with nature), are now encompassed by the term "spirituality." In this new sense, spirituality is the larger phenomenon, with religion reserved for that subset of spiritual phenomena that involve organized religious activity.

Such efforts to avoid the perceived stigma of "religion" shift all of its favored aspects to the old term, "spirituality." As a religious scholar, I must admit that I have mixed feelings about this development. "Religion" is a perfectly fine word, defined as the connection between humans and God. "Spirituality," too, is a fine word, with a precise usage agreed upon for centuries. But times change, as do the meanings of words. Rather than resist these changes, for purposes of clarity I have chosen to adopt these new usages. Throughout this book, where I refer to practices, beliefs, and experiences pertaining to organized religions or belief systems, I use the words "religion," "religious," and "religiousness." References to the domain of life beyond the body and mind make use of the words "spiritual" and "spirituality." Where I refer to the scientific field described in this book, I use either "religion" or "spirituality," or both.

Identifying "Active Ingredients" in Religion and Spirituality

Findings in the epidemiology of religion, like most epidemiologic research, describe the who, where, and when of a religion-health connection. These are important questions for scientists. But by itself, this information does not tell us what it is about religion and spirituality that benefits health, and how and why it does so. Saying that religion or spirituality is good for your health is like saying that eating food is good for your health. No doubt, if one were to conduct a long-term study of folks who eat and folks who do not eat at all, the ones who eat would, of course, be found to be healthier and live longer than the ones who starved themselves! But this fact alone would not give us a single clue as to what it is about eating that benefits health, what foods are good for us, or why. Most likely, some foods are good for our health and some are bad, with variations across different groups of people and across different situations.

Likewise, there are many types of religious practices and many ways of being spiritual. We need to examine their content to determine how and why they are connected with health and well-being. *God, Faith, and Health* asks these questions: What is it about religion and spirituality that is good for our health, and why is it so?

The first seven chapters of this book provide answers to these questions. Each chapter presents scientific evidence that a particular religious dimension or expression of spirituality benefits health and well-being, and then explains how it does so. This involves identifying the factors that explain the effects of religion on health. We know that a state of disease, or health, is rarely brought about by single factors that act directly and instantly. Rather, illness and wellness tend to develop over time, caused by multiple factors acting together. Likewise, spirituality works along with characteristics and functions of both body and mind to influence our health.

One way to look at these factors is as links in a chain between a potentially health-promoting factor, such as religion, and subsequent health and well-being. Each aspect or expression of spirituality described in this book benefits health through activating certain mental, emotional, or behavioral processes that we know promote health or prevent illness. Like the vitamins and nutrients in the food we eat, these factors are the "active ingredients" in our spiritual life. Identifying them helps us explain how and why religious involvement and spirituality influence our health.

Seven Principles of Theosomatic Medicine

This book takes a journey into deeper and more personal expressions of religion and spirituality. Each successive chapter discusses the health effects of increasingly "inner" types of spiritual expression. I begin with religious affiliation (Chapter 1) and move on to address active religious fellowship (Chapter 2), worship and prayer (Chapter 3), affirmation of religious beliefs (Chapter 4), profession of faith (Chapter 5), experience of mystical states of consciousness (Chapter 6), and finally, transcendent connection or union with God or the divine (Chapter 7).

Parallel to this journey is an exploration of more provocative and controversial scientific evidence on factors linking these types of spiritual expression to physical and mental health. Each successive chapter looks at the role of increasingly sophisticated factors at the cutting edge of science. I begin with healthy behavior (Chapter 1) and go on to consider social relationships (Chapter 2), the psychophysiology of emotions (Chapter 3), healthy beliefs and personality styles (Chapter 4), salutary thoughts and placebo effects (Chapter 5), altered states of consciousness and subtle energies (Chapter 6), and the possibility of supernatural influences (Chapter 7).

In each chapter, I offer some personal reflections. I also ask readers to consider the role of religion and spirituality in their own lives, and to reflect on how their beliefs or practices have influenced their health.

Each chapter looks thoroughly at a particular set of links among factors related to body, mind, and spirit, and includes a case history that illustrates the connections emphasized in the chapter. An opportunity is given to see these links in action, and to reflect on how they operate in one's life. By establishing and reflecting upon these links, we can identify seven guiding principles supported by research findings described in each chapter. These principles describe precisely the ways religion and spirituality benefit our health.

Part 1 explores the health benefits of the behavioral and social functions of religious expression. Chapters 1 and 2 describe how the public dimensions of religious participation—affiliation, membership, and attendance—work to prevent illness and promote health and well-being. These chapters help us to identify our first two guiding principles:

PRINCIPLE 1

Religious affiliation and membership benefit health by promoting healthy behavior and lifestyles.

PRINCIPLE 2

Regular religious fellowship benefits health by offering support that buffers the effects of stress and isolation.

Part 2 explores the psychological functions of spirituality. Chapters 3 through 5 describe how private expressions of spirituality engender emotions, beliefs, and thoughts that alleviate physical and psychological distress and promote good health. These chapters can be summarized in three more guiding principles:

PRINCIPLE 3

Participation in worship and prayer benefits health through the physiological effects of positive emotions.

PRINCIPLE 4

Religious beliefs benefit health by their similarity to health-promoting beliefs and personality styles.

PRINCIPLE 5

Simple faith benefits health by leading to thoughts of hope, optimism, and positive expectation.

Part 3 investigates concepts at the cutting edge of both spirituality and medical science. Chapter 6 examines the role of consciousness and subtle energies in the religion-and-health field—active ingredients or pathways considerably more controversial and provocative than those explored in the first five chapters. This discussion leads us to a sixth guiding principle:

PRINCIPLE 6

Mystical experiences benefit health by activating a healing bioenergy or life force or altered state of consciousness.

The first six chapters describe how religion and spirituality *promote health and prevent illness*. Chapter 7, by contrast, examines scientific evidence that certain spiritual practices, such as prayer for oneself or others, also play a role in the *healing of disease*—not just the prevention of illness. Several possible explanations for these provocative and controversial findings are offered. The information in this chapter supports a seventh guiding principle:

PRINCIPLE 7

Absent prayer for others is capable of healing by paranormal means or by divine intervention.

Chapter 8 envisions a future in which the scientific evidence presented here will be inextricably woven into both biomedical research and the practice of medicine. There is reason to believe that this will happen, and soon. The idea that body, mind, and spirit are in some way connected is an old one—almost universally accepted among religious traditions and systems of healing, except for the twentieth-century biomedicine of the Western world. But it is changing, thanks in part to the research described in *God, Faith, and Health*.

Awareness of a psychosomatic, or mind-body, connection has transformed psychology, medicine, science, and social institutions over the past few decades. Likewise, scientific evidence for connections among body, mind, and spirit promises to further expand the scientific worldview. A new perspective is gained from which the mind-body model seems almost as limited as the outdated, mechanistic, body-only model of contemporary medicine and science. I term this new perspective "theosomatic medicine"—literally, a model or view of the determinants of health based on the apparent connections between God, or spirit, and the body. This new-but-old vision of human life as a nexus of body, mind, and spirit offers the best way to make sense of exciting scientific findings and to shed new light on the mysteries of health and illness.

Let us now begin our journey through the seven principles of theosomatic medicine.

PART 1

The Health Effects of Public Religion

The religious impulse in human beings is expressed in many ways. One of these ways is through participation in organized public religious activities. The following two chapters explore the health benefits of public religious participation, with an emphasis on its behavioral and social functions. It is through its effect on our behavior and social relationships that public religious involvement works to prevent illness and promote health and well-being.

The evidence in these chapters supports the first two principles of theosomatic medicine:

PRINCIPLE 1

Religious affiliation and membership benefit health by promoting healthy behavior and lifestyles.

PRINCIPLE 2

Regular religious fellowship benefits health by offering support that buffers the effects of stress and isolation.

1

Religious Affiliation and a Healthy Lifestyle

Michael was never very good at taking care of his health, and he knew it. The owner of a small business, he was a workaholic and under a lot of stress. He smoked cigarettes, drank too much, ate poorly, and was overweight. Most of the time he was depressed and felt pretty lousy. Even though he knew he should mend his ways, nothing ever seemed to motivate him enough to change.

When the Persian Gulf War began, Michael's son was deployed. Michael loved his son and was very proud that he was serving his country, but the possibility of him dying thousands of miles away left Michael panicked. For the first time in his life, he turned to God. Although Michael had never considered himself religious and did not attend church, he had been raised in the Roman Catholic Church and was taught to believe in a God who answered prayers. Michael began to pray for his son to return home safely. He prayed fervently and constantly, many times a day, and offered God a deal. If God would ensure his son's safety, Michael would give religion a try and clean up his act.

Several weeks later, his son safely home, Michael honored his agreement with God. He renewed his connection with the Catholic Church. He started attending Mass, and soon began taking an active part in church activities. As he became more committed in his faith, Michael felt a burden to live more in accordance with Church teachings. He fulfilled his promise to God and quit drinking and stopped smoking cigarettes. It was not easy, but he had made a vow to God that he was determined not to break. Because he read in the Bible that the body is the temple of the Holy Spirit, he decided to improve his diet and to begin to exercise regularly. His health, and his spirits, improved dramatically.

Today Michael is a devout Catholic, surprisingly fit and healthy for a man of fifty. Although middle-aged, he looks much younger, and people are always surprised to discover that he has grown children. He has more energy than he ever did before, and a renewed outlook on life. His commitment to the teachings of his church inspire him to take better care of himself and to look for ways to help improve the health of others. He leads a full and active life, which now includes a daily run and regular Bible study.

We are a nation of religious believers. National surveys repeatedly show that about 90 percent of Americans, regardless of age, affiliate themselves with a religion or religious denomination. Not everyone who belongs to a religion is necessarily a member of a church, synagogue, or religious institution, or even regularly participates in services. Even among folks who are not religiously active, few choose the "none of the above" category in surveys about religious affiliation. The data are clear and consistent on one point: nearly all of us identify with a specific religion or belief system, whether we are involved in the practice of religion as prescribed in its teachings or not.

All religions promote belief systems known as doctrines. Some religions or denominations contain hundreds of doctrines that adherents are supposed to endorse. These shared beliefs are expected to shape the behavior of believers, guiding their conduct in life situations. In *Dimensions of the Sacred*, Dr. Ninian Smart, professor of comparative religions at the University of California, categorizes many of the issues typically addressed in such doctrines. These issues include:

1. the existence of God or a supreme being,
2. the characteristics of this being,
3. the presence of other supernatural beings such as angels,
4. our relationship with God and the supernatural realm,
5. the creation of the universe and of human beings,
6. the nature of space and time,
7. the existence of the soul,
8. what happens to humans and human souls when their carnal bodies die,
9. the way or path that we must follow to attain salvation or redemption or to reach heaven or paradise, and
10. the nature of reality.

Most religions or denominations throughout the world offer statements of belief regarding these issues and others, and diverse faiths often endorse similar beliefs. The doctrines of Protestants, Catholics, Jews, and Muslims testify to the existence of an all-powerful God who created the universe several thousand years ago. On other questions, such as what to do or believe in order to be redeemed or saved or to be rewarded with eternal life, religions differ widely.

For example, evangelical Christians affirm that salvation is granted through what theologians refer to as "vicarious atonement." Salvation is attained through God's grace when people surrender their lives to Jesus Christ, whose death and resurrection wipes away the sins of those who accept him as Lord and Savior. Jewish tradition, by contrast, holds that individual Jews are duty-bound whenever possible to observe *mitzvot*—the 613 commandments described in the Torah (Old Testament) and required of the faithful. Some commandments are positive ("thou shalt") and some are negative ("thou shalt not"); but all Jews, it is held, are accountable to God for their observance. In the orthodox Hindu system of Brahmanism, the concept of salvation itself takes on an entirely different meaning. All human souls are subject to *samsara*, an eternal cycle of death and rebirth, until a state of such purity is attained that the soul transcends the need for further incarnation.

Clearly, not only do religious doctrines cover a broad range of human concerns, but for particular issues, they may vary widely across religions or religious denominations. For individuals who identify with a particular faith tradition, their affirmation or rejection of such doctrines has a lot to say about how they live their lives. One's commitment to religious doctrines can influence almost any area of life.

Religious Beliefs about Healthy Behavior

In a review that my colleagues and I recently published in a leading public health journal, we identified behaviors and attitudes related to many areas of life that studies have shown are influenced by people's commitment to their religion. That is, the more or less religiously committed one is, the more or less likely one is to engage in particular behaviors or profess certain attitudes. Areas that might be affected include political preference and voting, sexual activity, criminal violations, contraceptive usage, patterns of social and interpersonal relationships, childbearing, marital happiness, and feelings about social issues such as the environment. Studies have shown that affiliation with a religion and commitment to particular religious doctrines can predict the way that people respond to questions about their preferences. For sociologists and other scientists who study these issues, this is old news.

What is not old news, and what may come as a surprise to many people—medical professionals and laypeople alike—is that considerable scientific evidence now shows that the influence of religious affiliation and commitment also extends to an unexpected area of human life: health.

According to Dr. Rachel E. Spector, author of *Cultural Diversity in Health and Illness*, nearly every religion espouses beliefs that govern behavior regarding health, disease, and death. Some beliefs *prescribe*, or require, behaviors related to health, and others *proscribe*, or forbid, behaviors related to health or medical care. For religiously committed people, many of the doctrines or teachings of their faith offer moral and practical guidance regarding how to attain, maintain, or recover physical and emotional health and well-being.

For example, Roman Catholic teachings forbid abortion and birth control. Jehovah's Witnesses eschew blood transfusions. Latter-Day Saints (Mormons) prohibit drinks such as tea and coffee. Christian Scientists typically refuse medical treatment from physicians. Jews, Hindus, Muslims, and Seventh-Day Adventists require, encourage, or discourage certain food choices. Other religions promote beliefs governing behaviors such as smoking, drinking, drug use, diet, sexual practices, general hygiene, and the use of medical care. For all religious traditions, the behavioral guidelines canonized in specific doctrines are there to provide committed believers with a road map that will point the way to, if not ensure, the kind of long and productive life that is thought to result from living in harmony with nature and nature's laws.

The Religious Factor in Health

As epidemiologic findings bear out, there is considerable wisdom in these behavioral guidelines.

I have already told the story of my discovery as a young graduate student of about two hundred published studies of religious differences in rates of health, illness, and death. Many of these studies were obscure and uncited by other scientists, and while finding them was a challenging task that took several years, sifting through them and trying to make sense of their findings was much easier. Study after study pointed to a common conclusion: religious affiliation, whatever the religion, seemed to be associated with lower rates of disease and death, whatever the cause of illness. In the special language used by epidemiologists, lack of religious affiliation was apparently a new and potent risk factor for ill health, across the board.

This was a startling finding. It was not something that I was ever taught as a graduate student in public health, and it is not usually taught to medical students or residents today. Yet the results are present and in great abundance. Further, while medical research findings are often ambiguous and tentative, the presence of a significant and salutary (health-promoting) religious factor is by now a consistent and expected finding in epidemiologic studies.

Evidence of a benefit of religious affiliation for health is supported for many diseases and conditions. Studies suggest that commitment to religion, expressed as affiliation with or membership in a denomination or particular church or synagogue, may have a protective effect against subsequent illness. Just as with refraining from cigarettes or alcohol or overeating, religious affiliation may prevent or delay pathogenic (illness-making) changes and have long-term benefits for physical and mental functioning and health.

Religion and Heart Disease

We identified more than fifty studies in which religious differences had been found in relation to a remarkable range of heart–disease–related conditions: death due to circulatory system diseases; arteriosclerotic heart disease incidence and death; myocardial infarction incidence and death; coronary artery disease prevalence; atherosclerosis prevalence; coronary heart disease incidence, prevalence, and death; rheumatic, nonrheumatic, and hypertensive heart disease death; angina pectoris incidence; aortic calcification prevalence; death due to chronic endocarditis; and incidence of numerous risk factors, such as high cholesterol, lipids, caloric and fat intake, and triglycerides.

For some religious groups, we observed an especially strong advantage:

- Scientists at the Missouri Center for Health Statistics found that the death rate due to ischemic heart disease in members of the Reorganized Church of Jesus Christ of Latter-Day Saints (RLDS) was only about 80 percent of that of other Missourians.
- Investigators at the University of Colorado, Case Western Reserve University, and Johns Hopkins University studied death rate patterns in the Old Order Amish people of Indiana, Ohio, and Pennsylvania. Males ages forty to sixty-nine had a 35 percent lower rate of death due to circulatory system diseases than non-Amish males of the same age.
- A team from the University of Utah found that Mormons had a death rate due to ischemic heart disease that was 35 percent lower than in non-Mormons. There were also Mormon advantages for deaths from hypertensive and rheumatic heart disease.
- Researchers from the Institute for Social Medicine in Utrecht found, for deaths caused by ischemic heart disease, an advantage of 57 percent for Seventh-Day Adventists, relative to non-Adventists.

Religion and Blood Pressure

We also identified many studies of religious differences in systolic and diastolic blood pressure and rates of hypertension. This serious illness has been subject to greater study and scrutiny with respect to religion than any other disease. So many studies have been conducted in this area that we felt a need existed to summarize these findings in a detailed review, which was published in the British journal *Social Science and Medicine*.

Among Seventh-Day Adventists, one of the religious groups found to have less heart disease, there is a history of less hypertension—including lower systolic and diastolic blood pressure—than among non-Adventists, in both sexes and most age groups. In one Australian study, which defined hypertension liberally as systolic and diastolic readings above 160 mmHg and 95 mmHg, respectively, 4.5 and 7.1 percent of non-Adventists reported a history of hypertension. Among Adventists, rates were only 2.6 and 2.3 percent.

Affiliation with other religious groups also results in distinct blood pressure advantages. A California study of adults with Chinese, Filipino, or Japanese ancestry found a 29.3 percent rate of hypertension in religiously nonaffiliated people. This was *twice* that of the religiously affiliated, whose rate was only 15.0 percent. Among Buddhists, hypertension was even less prevalent: 10.9 percent.

A famous study from the Harvard School of Public Health examined hypertension in South African Zulus. Results were quite unusual. Among urban women, membership in a Christian church was associated with normal blood pressure; nonmembers were more likely to have hypertension. Nonmembership coupled with occult involvement had further consequences: urban women who reported being the object of sorcery had greater hypertension. A follow-up study found high blood pressure more than twice as prevalent among women who reported being "bewitched."

When it comes to high blood pressure, the advantage ascribed to religious affiliation even extends to the religious commitment of one's relatives. This is what Israeli researchers found in a study of blood pressure among Jewish families in Jerusalem. Among female children, regardless of their own religious activity, having a father who attended yeshiva (received formal Jewish religious training) for at least five years was dramatically protective. These youngsters had a mean diastolic blood pressure of 65.2 mmHg. Those whose father had one to four years of Yeshiva had an average reading *nearly 10 points higher*: 74.5 mmHg. Those having a father with no religious training had a diastolic blood pressure somewhere in between: 71.5. Apparently, as to the health benefits of being raised by a father with a formal Jewish education, an incomplete education is worse than no Jewish training at all.

The Clergy and Hypertension

One group of people has, by definition, a much higher than average rate of religious affiliation and membership: the clergy. How does their blood pressure compare to that of the rest of the population? Remarkably well, and their particular religion or denomination does not seem to matter.

When researchers from the National Cancer Institute and Georgetown University compared death rates in American Baptist clergymen to those in the general Caucasian population of the United States, ministers were almost *40 percent less likely* to die of hypertension complicated by heart disease. Limiting analysis to twenty- to sixty-four-year-olds yielded an even more remarkable *66 percent advantage*. Compared to all men with work experience (avoiding the bias of including men too sick to have ever worked), there is an astounding *82 percent advantage*. Compared to all other Caucasian clergymen, these Baptist ministers still do better: a 74 percent advantage. But pastors of other denominations need not worry: compared to the general population, they have mortality advantages for hypertension of 29 percent (Presbyterians) to as high as 41 percent (Lutherans and Episcopalians).

The blood pressure advantages of pastoring extend beyond Christian clergy in the United States. Japanese scientists conducted a fascinating study of mortality among priests of the Myoshinji branch of the Rinzai sect of Zen Buddhism. They examined nearly two dozen diseases and conditions, and the most striking finding was for death due to hypertensive diseases. Compared to other Japanese men, priests were exactly *half as likely* to die from hypertension. The health benefits of ordination are no respecter, it seems, of what religion you choose—as long as you choose one.

Religion and Cancer

Dozens of studies report religious differences in rates of cancer, both overall and for many specific types of cancer. As with heart disease and hypertension, affiliation with certain religions or denominations offers considerable protection.

Studies conducted at UCLA, the University of Utah, and the University of Alberta revealed a lower overall death rate in Mormons, from the 1950s through 1970s, in both sexes, in Utah, California, and Canada. Moreover, Mormons are protected *not just from dying of cancer but from getting cancer*, in both sexes, overall and for many cancer sites.

Studies conducted at Loma Linda University School of Public Health likewise have identified lower death rates for Seventh-Day Adventists overall and for several cancer sites, including colon, rectum, lung, and mouth. As with Mormons, Adventists are also protected from getting cancer.

Seventh-Day Adventists are protected in other ways. Research from the prestigious Sloan-Kettering Institute found fewer than expected numbers of hospital cases of cancer in Adventists. A study from the Danish Cancer Registry showed a significant advantage in Adventist men for cancers of the colon, respiratory system, and bladder. Adventist women also have an advantage in survival following diagnosis with breast cancer. An Indiana University study summarized thirty years of data from California and found higher one-, three-, five-, and ten-year survival rates in Adventists.

Mormons and Seventh-Day Adventists are not alone in experiencing a relative advantage in rates of cancer incidence and death. The Hutterite Brethren are a small Christian sect that resides in communal agricultural colonies in North America. They are organized in three nonintermarrying subgroups known as Dariusleut, Lehrerleut, and Schmiedeleut. Hutterites are interesting for epidemiologists to study because they are so isolated and homogeneous both genetically and in terms of lifestyle.

Scientists at Northwestern University found fewer than expected cancer deaths for Hutterites in South Dakota and Manitoba. They also found advantages for cancer deaths overall and at several sites. A study from the University of Alberta found that this Hutterite advantage in cancer mortality also extends to morbidity. Over a twenty-year period, Hutterites in Canada developed fewer than expected new cases of cancer, overall and at several sites.

Jews and Cancer

Of special interest to researchers has been the relative advantage of Jews for certain cancers. Documentation of a protective effect of Jewish identity for reproductive cancers, such as of the uterus or cervix, or for cancers of the male organs, dates to the early nineteenth century, when Dr. Benjamin Travers noted never having seen a case of penile cancer in a Jew. Scholarly articles published early in the twentieth century noted especially lower rates of uterine and cervical cancer in Jewish women. This was attributed to the hygienic benefit of circumcision in their partners. The assumption was made that Jewish women were more likely to engage Jewish (circumcised) men as sexual partners, which would lower their risk for cancers that were more likely, on average, to be found in uncircumcised men. Lending credence to this assumption is research showing an enormously higher incidence of penile cancer in Hindus, who are not typically circumcised, relative to Muslims, who are, and in whom such cancers are almost unheard of.

The first half of the twentieth century saw many studies of religious differences in these cancers. Much of this work was reviewed in 1948 by Dr. E. L. Kennaway of St. Bartholomew's Hospital in London. Dr. Kennaway examined data on uterine cancer in Jewish women from five U.S. cities, seven European countries, and the area then known as Palestine. He also examined data from Hindus, Muslims, Parsis, and Indian Christians, as well as Chinese women. His findings distinctly revealed fewer new cases of cancer in Jews relative to gentiles and in Parsis relative to Hindus. The total current cases of cancer were fewer in Muslims than in Hindus.

Since Dr. Kennaway's summary, many epidemiologic studies have confirmed that some religious groups do better than others. My own files on this topic number more than fifty studies published into the 1990s. Across these studies, the protected groups—the religious groups whose members seem to be at lower risk of uterine or cervical cancer—are by now familiar: Mormons, Seventh-Day Adventists, Hutterites, Amish, Muslims, Parsis, and Jews. When compared to population groups of "all others," women affiliated with these groups, especially Jewish women, have lower incidence (new cases), prevalence (total cases), and mortality.

For certain other cancer sites that are unrelated, one presumes, to a hypothetical public-health benefit of circumcision, Jews also have considerably lower rates.

- A Dutch study from over fifty years ago found fewer than expected deaths among Jews from cancers of the stomach and bile passages.
- A study conducted at the University of Texas Medical Branch found, over a fifteen-year period, an average annual death rate due to lung cancer in gentile men of 148.6 per 100,000; in Jewish men the rate was 92.5 per 100,000—*more than 60 percent lower.*
- Reviewing data sources from studies conducted in New York City, Dr. William Haenszel of the National Cancer Institute found lower rates of death in Jews relative to non-Jews for cancers of the buccal cavity, pharynx, prostate, and bladder.

Religion, Health, and Death

Many other studies focus on how religious affiliation affects the overall morbidity or mortality of a population, be it a particular community or an entire nation. Epidemiologists consider the total mortality rate and its counterpart, life expectancy at birth, to be reliable indicators of a population's health. Illness indices, such as self-ratings of overall health, reported histories of chronic diseases, and counts of particular symptoms, are also useful indicators of the general health of a group of people.

By now, it should be no surprise to discover the protected groups:

- In U.S., European, and Australian studies, Seventh-Day Adventists have fewer respiratory symptoms, better cardiovascular health, less mortality, and higher life expectancy.
- RLDS Mormons in Missouri and Utah have greater life expectancy relative to non-Mormons, overall, in both sexes, and in nearly all age groups.
- Researchers have studied death rates among the Amish in Indiana, Ohio, and Pennsylvania. For Amish females between

the ages of ten and thirty-nine, there is a 34 percent advantage. For men aged forty to sixty-nine, the advantage is even greater: 39 percent.

- Studies dating to the 1950s describe a similar Jewish advantage. In New York City, for example, Jews have a lower all-causes death rate at all ages.

Another group of studies suggests that the benefits of religious affiliation for overall rates of illness and death are no respecter of what religion one endorses. Simply affiliating with a religion or joining a religious institution, in general, compared to not affiliating at all, offers a distinct advantage.

- In a follow-up study of nearly 7,000 Californians surveyed nine years earlier, nonmembership in a church—any church—increased the risk of death by 1.4 times, in both sexes. This magnitude of risk was comparable to that of infrequent use of health care, high alcohol consumption, inactivity, and obesity.
- Using data from the 1972–1977 General Social Survey of the National Opinion Research Center, researchers found that regardless of one's religion or denomination, those who simply acknowledged being a "strong," as opposed to "not so strong," affiliate of a religion were more satisfied with their health.
- In data from the 1984 General Social Survey, those who reported being strongly affiliated with a religion—any religion—were more likely to rate themselves as very happy and very satisfied with their family life, and to find life exciting.

How Extensive Is the Religion-Health Connection?

In case this selection of findings from our original review of about two hundred studies is still not convincing, consider the following. When I give presentations on this topic to medical groups or at scientific meetings, I often show a few slides that document the amazing breadth of scientific findings that point to religious differences in rates of disease. Across the hundreds of studies that have by now investigated such differences, at least one study somewhere has uncovered a significant religious difference in relation to the following illnesses or conditions:

allergies/hay fever
angina pectoris
asthma
atherosclerosis
back pain
benign gynecological disorders
bronchitis/persistent
    cough
cancer pain
coronary artery disease
coronary heart disease
digestive diseases
early menopause
emphysema

epinephrinelike
    cardiovascular pattern
family history of diabetes
family history of stroke
hypertension
illness symptoms
myocardial infarction
pneumonia/influenza
regional enteritis
self-rated health
trichomoniasis
tuberculosis
tuberculin test sensitivity
    ulcerative colitis

Likewise, at least one study somewhere has uncovered a significant religious difference in relation to the following causes of death:

accidents/violence
angina pectoris
asthma
atherosclerosis
bronchitis/respiratory diseases
coronary artery disease
coronary heart disease
circulatory system diseases
central nervous system diseases
cerebrovascular disease
diabetes
digestive diseases
duodenal or peptic ulcer
emphysema

endocrine/metabolic disorders
genitourinary diseases
hypertension/stroke
infant mortality
kidney disease
liver disease
myocardial infarction
nonrheumatic chronic
    endocarditis
pneumonia/influenza/
    infectious diseases
prostate hyperplasia
syphilis
tuberculosis

For the following types of cancer:

bladder/kidney	ovaries
brain/central nervous system	pancreas
breast	penis
bucca	pharynx
cervix	prostate
colon/small intestine	rectum
esophagus	skin
larynx	stomach
leukemia/lymphomas	tongue
lip	uterus
liver/gallbladder	vulva/vagina
lung/bronchus/trachea	

For deaths from the following types of cancer:

bladder/urinary tract	lymphomas
bone	ovaries/fallopian tubes
brain/central nervous system	pancreas
breast	peritoneum
bucca/lip/tongue	penis
cervix	pharynx
colon	prostate
digestive system	rectum
esophagus	skin
eye	small intestine
Hodgkin's	stomach
kidney	testicles/scrotum
larynx	thyroid/endocrine system
leukemia	uterus
liver/gallbladder/bile duct	vulva/vagina/clitoris
lung/bronchus/trachea	

Among the protected populations throughout these studies, the same religious groups keep coming up: Amish, Buddhist priests, Catholic nuns, church members in general, Hindus, Hutterites, Jains, Jews, Latter-Day Saints, Muslims, Reorganized Latter-Day Saints, Parsis, Protestant clergy, Seventh-Day Adventists, and Trappist monks.

What do these religious groups have in common?

While we find striking differences in health and illness across religions, the most favorable results are among members of religions that make strict behavioral demands. Less favorable results appear in those with other affiliations or none at all. Demands typically involve prescribed and proscribed actions in relation to health, such as regulating diet, physical activity, sexuality, and tobacco and alcohol use.

Links in a Chain:
Religious Affiliation→Healthy Behavior→Health

Why are religiously affiliated people healthier, on average, than the less religiously committed? This is a complicated question, and epidemiologists and medical scientists have not yet come up with an answer that is conclusively proven to everyone's satisfaction. In light of what we know about how religious commitment influences behavior and how behavior influences health, a reasonable answer can be proposed. I believe that it is the behaviorally prescriptive and proscriptive nature of religious commitment that best accounts for the more favorable health profile of religiously affiliated people.

For sure, while not all religiously affiliated people follow all of the health-related guidelines of their particular faith, we can expect that, on average, people who report a religious identity are more likely to follow the dictates of their religion than people who report no affiliation at all. Among these religiously affiliated and committed people, commitment to health-promoting religious doctrines encourages healthy practices that prevent illness and enhance physical and emotional health and overall well-being. Can this be proven?

If we think of the relationships among religious affiliation, healthy behavior, and health as links on a chain, then to support my assertion, we need to examine the research evidence for two of these links: from religious affiliation to healthy behavior, and from healthy behavior to health. As I will show, research findings support both of these links. Considerable research shows that membership in particular religions or religious denominations correlates strongly with the practice of healthy behavior. This is a familiar finding to researchers in the fields of medical sociology and the sociology of religion. Additional findings from epidemiologic studies show that unhealthy behaviors are associated with higher rates of disease and death. This is one of the most commonly observed findings in the fields of social and behavioral epidemiology. Together, these findings establish the link between religious affiliation and health, and support the conclusion that religious involvement should be considered a vital component of a healthy lifestyle.

Religious Affiliation and a Healthy Lifestyle: Two Sides of the Same Coin?

Just as research points to religious differences in health, so, too, do studies identify religious differences in the kinds of behaviors that determine our health. Not surprisingly, the religious groups with the most favorable health profiles are also the groups that most actively and explicitly promote healthy behavioral choices and healthy living in general.

- Mormons are much less likely to smoke tobacco or drink alcohol, consume caffeinated beverages such as coffee or tea, or have multiple sexual partners. Each of these behaviors is a known risk factor for cancer.
- Seventh-Day Adventists are more likely to abstain from tobacco and alcohol and to follow a lacto-ovo-vegetarian diet, choices that protect against cancer. Adventists who are stricter in their observance of dietary guidelines also have lower rates of death due to heart disease.
- The Amish and Hutterites discourage tobacco use, discourage alcohol use or tolerate it only in moderation, and exhibit very low levels of premarital and extramarital sex. These factors are responsible, in part, for their lower rates of cancer.

A connection between religious involvement and healthy behavior, at least in principle, is obvious. No major religion openly encourages sloth, promiscuity, drunkenness, drug abuse, and obesity. But not all of us do such a good job in following the dictates of our religion. Still, a link between religious involvement and healthy behavior is apparent. Surveying results of behavioral and epidemiologic studies, noted religious scholar Dr. Kenneth Vaux concluded: "It appears that religious beliefs and associated moral habits vitally affect health attitudes and behaviors. As a result of this causal relationship, health and disease indices vary in important ways according to the penetration of these beliefs into the daily fabric of the patient's life." Dr. Vaux explained that religious participation and exposure to religious beliefs predispose us to act in ways that profoundly affect our health. Religions may wrap a blanket of moral sanction around certain behaviors that directly or indirectly influence physical health and emotional well-being.

Religious Prescriptions and Proscriptions

Certain behavioral prescriptions and proscriptions are almost universally promoted by religious groups. These include avoidance of smoking and drug use, moderation in or abstinence from alcohol consumption, specific dietary restrictions, regulations regarding cleanliness and hygiene, and forbiddance of sexual promiscuity. The potential health benefits are obvious. These are the exact same behaviors identified as the most important targets of health promotion efforts by scientists in key government reports on the nation's health.

Besides these obviously health-related behaviors promoted by almost all religions, Dr. Vaux identified other healthy behaviors that are encouraged by the moral codes of particular religions. These include the following activities: (1) exercising and maintaining physical fitness, (2) meditating, (3) getting enough sleep, (4) being vaccinated, (5) being willing to have the body examined, (6) undertaking a pilgrimage for health reasons, (7) telling the truth about how you feel, (8) maintaining family viability, (9) hoping for recovery, (10) coping with stress, (11) undergoing genetic screening and counseling, (12) being able to live with a handicap, and (13) caring for children.

Studies have identified religious differences in other behaviors known to affect our health. Many of these studies point to a distinct advantage among Jews in the performance of healthy behaviors and avoidance of risky behaviors. Examples include less frequent use of mouthwash; more frequent preventive medical behavior; and greater likelihood of having received a diagnostic X-ray and of visiting a physician, taking medications, and staying home when ill.

Studies identifying religious differences in rates of health care use are another little-known area of health research that my collegues and I reviewed several years ago. In a paper published in the British journal *Social Science and Medicine*, we summarized results of over thirty such studies. We found evidence of religious differences in immunization, psychiatric care utilization, use of maternal and child health services, dental care, hospitalization, and physician visits. We concluded that affiliation with a religion increases one's exposure to religious beliefs that serve, on average, to encourage and reinforce healthy practices, including seeking necessary preventive care and medical treatment.

Doing Better and Feeling Worse: Does Our Behavior Influence Our Health?

In the mid-1970s, the president of the Rockefeller Foundation, Dr. John H. Knowles, organized a group of scientists to study health care problems and make recommendations for public policy. Dr. Knowles convened a group of highly respected experts, scholarly papers were solicited, and many of the final drafts were gathered together and published in a volume of *Daedalus*, the official journal of the American Academy of Arts and Sciences. This material was published in 1977 as a popular book, *Doing Better and Feeling Worse*. This title reflected the conclusions of many of the panelists that despite the availability of the technologically finest medical care in the world, Americans were less satisfied than ever with their care. Worse, significant pockets of citizens—the poor, children, the elderly, ethnic minorities—were doing less well than other groups. Further, certain of the so-called diseases of civilization—chronic, degenerative diseases such as heart disease, cancer, and hypertension—were responsible for a greater proportion of illness than ever before.

In "The Responsibility of the Individual," Dr. Knowles described how improvements in environmental conditions related to food production, milk and water safety, and sewage disposal helped to diminish the scourge of communicable disease that plagued the developed world into the early decades of the twentieth century. The greater importance during that period of advances in sanitation and hygiene over the relatively less prominent role of medical care in dramatically improving the life expectancy of Americans is well known by all public health professionals. As death rates declined, Knowles continued, medicine became overconfident, asserting that high-tech diagnostic and therapeutic innovations were all that was needed to usher in an era of perfect health for all. Clearly, this utopian vision has failed. The culprit, he asserted, was our personal behavior.

Dr. Knowles's thesis was that the key to the health of a nation is for individuals to avoid behaviors that put their health at risk. For policy makers, cultivating "individual responsibility" for health was just a matter of finding the right message, then repeating it and reinforcing it through peer pressure. "Advertising agencies know this," Dr. Knowles added, but he admitted the difficulty in selling the public on health. Nevertheless, the answer was simple: "The individual has the power—indeed, the moral responsibility—to maintain his own health by the observance of simple, prudent rules of behavior relating to sleep, exercise, diet and weight, alcohol, and smoking. In addition, he should avoid where possible the long-term use of drugs."

While Dr. Knowles's prescription for public-health policy remains controversial, his diagnosis of particular behaviors or lifestyles as much ignored by scientifically verified determinants of health and illness is absolutely sound. According to a report issued by the Institute of Medicine, "50% of mortality from the 10 leading causes of death in the U.S. can be traced to lifestyle." This "burden of illness" due to behavior is reflected in death and illness statistics, as well as in rates of disability, job days lost, and hospitalization. Health-destroying behavior is a factor in the incidence of heart disease, cancer, hypertension, diabetes, respiratory diseases, cirrhosis of the liver, and other chronic illnesses. These facts led prominent health psychologist Dr. Joseph M. Matarazzo to propose that smoking, drinking, overeating, and the like constitute "behavioral pathogens." That is, these behaviors are as qualified to be considered direct, disease-causing agents as any virus, bacterium, or other microorganism.

Healthy Behavior and Social Ties: The Alameda County Study

The best-known epidemiologic study of the impact of behavior on longevity and subsequent rates of illness is the Alameda County Study. In 1965, investigators in Berkeley, California, surveyed nearly 7,000 adults, inquiring about their medical history and current health as well as a very extensive range of issues related to health practices, family life, social activities, interests, and feelings and attitudes. Every few years, this original cohort of respondents (those who respond to a survey) is reinterviewed.

This type of study has allowed scientists to investigate the long-term health effects of certain personal characteristics. A longitudinal or prospective study design is much sought after by epidemiologists, because it enables us to dispense with the chicken-or-egg quandary in attributing higher rates of illness to certain causes. It is different from a cross-sectional study—one in which questions about health and exposures or potential risk factors are asked all at the same time and only once. Without follow-up, one can never be fully certain just what caused what. Did alcohol consumption lead to cirrhosis of the liver, or did a diagnosis of cirrhosis drive sick people to drink?

Findings from the Alameda County Study form the foundation of behavioral epidemiology, the study of how behavior influences health and illness. Published analyses of these data helped to publicize the famous "seven healthy practices" familiar to (but certainly not followed by) most adult Americans. These include: (1) getting seven to eight hours of sleep every night, (2) eating breakfast every day, (3) rarely eating between meals, (4) remaining near one's ideal weight, (5) never smoking, (6) avoiding or being moderate in use of alcohol, and (7) getting regular physical activity. Numerous publications since have determined that current observance of these healthy behaviors, alone or in tandem, is a strong predictor of rates of health and illness, often many years later.

One of the most interesting studies to come from the Alameda County data was described in the scientific article, "Social Networks, Host Resistance, and Mortality," published in the prestigious *American Journal of Epidemiology* in 1979. The article was written by Drs. Lisa F. Berkman and S. Leonard Syme, two of the world's most respected social epidemiologists. Their study found that individuals with strong social ties, including membership in a church or synagogue, had significantly lower death rates than those without such connections. One might think these findings on the health benefits of strong social relationships belong in the next chapter, "Religious Fellowship and Spiritual Support," except for one very curious and very exceptional finding.

Dr. Berkman, now chairperson of the Department of Health and Social Behavior at the Harvard School of Public Health, and Dr. Syme, currently emeritus professor of epidemiology at the University of California, described this finding in painstaking detail. One's standing on a scale of social network ties, including religious membership, had a direct effect on longevity *even after taking into account* the mortality-increasing effects of several harmful behaviors: smoking, drinking, obesity, physical inactivity, and infrequent preventive care. What does this imply? Just this: although each of these behaviors increases the risk of death, and while each is less common in those with more social ties, the longevity-increasing impact of social ties such as religion persist regardless of the harmful effects of these behaviors.

Although destructive health practices indeed have harmful effects on health—this cannot be denied—the findings of Berkman and Syme demonstrated that these behaviors do not occur in a vacuum. They are influenced by other factors, including religious group membership, whose own health effects seem to extend above and beyond their ability to influence behavior. This by now is well established. But it is the protective effect of religious affiliation for health, especially through its effects on behavior, that deserves greater consideration. Membership in churches and synagogues—institutions that prescribe and proscribe certain behaviors—reflects a level of religious commitment that may have a lot to say about how often people smoke, drink, abuse drugs, and do or do not take care of themselves in ways that can prolong or cut short their lives.

Lessons to Consider

The evidence in this chapter gives rise to the first of our seven principles of theosomatic medicine:

PRINCIPLE 1

Religious affiliation and membership benefit health by promoting healthy behavior and lifestyles

---

What can we learn from scientific studies linking religious affiliation to better health through the promotion of healthy behavior? What do these findings mean for us as individuals? What conclusions can we draw?

Just as health varies according to other personal characteristics—age, gender, ethnic background, marital status, socioeconomic status, and so on—so, too, does health vary by religious affiliation. From the overview of published findings, we know that certain religious groups do better than others when it comes to disease and death. Members of religious groups that put restrictions on certain detrimental behaviors, or offer guidelines or encouragement supportive of healthy behavior, are at decreased risk of heart disease, hypertension, and cancer, and seem to live longer and to be in better health.

While affiliation with a religion or membership in a denomination or church obviously does not guarantee us perfect health—nothing can do that—it may increase our exposure to health-promoting messages and to friends who maintain healthy lifestyles sanctioned by official religious teachings. It bears repeating here that epidemiologic findings are generalizations. They are based on relationships between risk factors and health outcomes that exist on average, across groups of people. We can always identify glaring exceptions—the chain-smoker who never gets lung cancer, the vegetarian marathon runner who drops dead at forty from heart disease—but these do not invalidate the overall association. Most of us recognize that if we smoke or are obese or do not get any exercise, we are increasing our risk of a serious illness. Sure, we may end up being one of the lucky ones who beat the odds—who fail to practice healthy behavior yet avoid chronic disease and early death. But I would bet that most of us are not willing to take that chance, especially when a healthy lifestyle not only decreases our health risks but helps us feel so good as well.

Is One Religion as Good as Another?

Sometimes, after lecturing about this research to a group of scientists or physicians, I am asked, in all seriousness, "So, what religion should I convert to in order to guarantee the best health?" The answer, of course, is that this question is unanswerable. All religions endorse the idea that we ought to take care of our bodies and not act in ways that are reckless and endanger our health. Affiliated members are free to ignore these teachings or take them to heart. In some faith traditions, however, the respect shown for health goes beyond lip service. It may represent a key focus of their teachings. What epidemiologic findings show is that being a part of a religious group or community that respects and honors the biblical idea that "your body is a temple of the Holy Spirit within you, which you have from God" (I Corinthians 6:19) increases the likelihood that somewhere along the way such messages will have "taken," and will have motivated healthy behavior.

You need not convert to a behaviorally strict religious denomination to improve your health or prolong your life. First of all, it is unlikely to work unless you take that religion's teachings on smoking, drinking, diet, sexuality, and the like seriously. And you hardly need to change your religion to do that. Second, choosing or affirming a spiritual path is one of life's most important decisions. There are an awful lot of reasons to affiliate with or join or convert to a particular religious group, and it is hard to imagine that favorable epidemiologic data belong at the top of the list. Affirming a particular religious identity ought to be for reasons of the soul.

What these findings suggest, though—strongly—is that religious affiliation may present the opportunity for potentially long-term benefits to your health and well-being above and beyond the more obvious benefit to your soul. When we place ourselves in situations where healthy living and responsible behavior are encouraged and supported, we are more likely to live that way ourselves, or at least try. Hearing positive health messages and seeing healthy lifestyles modeled make it easier to adopt such ways of living. This can occur through affiliation with more conservative religious groups or membership in more religiously observant congregations or through ascetic vows. But it can also occur through joining a hatha yoga class, or convening a group of friends to meet regularly for meditation, or participating in a study group of the teachings of Edgar Cayce or Rudolf Steiner, or being part of a Jewish Renewal *chavurah*. It is a fact of life that when we affiliate with other people following a specific spiritual path, it becomes easier to follow that path.

Questions to Reflect On

At the beginning of this chapter, I talked about Michael. At a crossroads in his life, he decided to actively affiliate with a church and to accept its teachings as guideposts for living. This resulted not only in a renewed sense of faith, but in a greater sense of overall well-being, physically and emotionally.

Michael's story is not unique Many of us come to a point in life when we choose to commit, or recommit, to a spiritual path. While few if any of us do so with health explicitly in mind, there may be unexpected health-related benefits of religious membership, especially if we begin affirming a new set of beliefs or values. Committing to a faith tradition or spiritual path presents an opportunity to explore new teachings, both official scriptures or doctrines and commentaries by learned figures. As discussed earlier, many of the teachings of the major religions have much to say about healthy living, and often recommend specific health-promoting practices. Choosing to follow a certain religious or spiritual path often means changing one's life in ways that ultimately may offer physical and emotional benefits. I know this to be true in my own life.

When I returned in earnest to my Jewish roots in my late twenties, I felt a hunger inside to learn all that I could about Jewish living. Slowly I started to incorporate more and more elements of a

Jewish lifestyle. These included changing how I ate, how I approached taking care of my body, how I viewed sexual matters, how much rest I got, how I spent my weekends, how I made a living, how I interacted with other people, and how I managed stress. Gone were the barhopping, social drinking, late nights, rich foods, sloth, excess weight, hanging out with the wrong people, and generally undisciplined and self-centered lifestyle of a committed bachelor. Motivated by a desire to live more in accord with *mitzvot*, or commandments, the guideposts to Jewish life, I began to reconnect with organized Judaism. Since then I have experienced tangible and positive changes in my physical functioning, my energy level, and my emotional equilibrium. I believe that my wife, my family, and my friends would agree.

If you are newly affiliated with a particular religion or religious denomination, or have recently recommitted or converted, you may be experiencing similar changes in the way you live your life. Likewise, if you have taken up a new spiritual path, such as pursuing meditation or following the teachings of a spiritual master or group, you may be in the process of changing what you value and therefore how you act. If you are a lifelong member of a particular faith, perhaps you recognize how your identification with that tradition has shaped your behavior. Several questions can help us reflect on how our religious or spiritual commitments have helped shape the actions that we take with respect to our health.

- What do the teachings of your religion or spiritual path have to say about the human body? Is it something to be cherished, perhaps as a receptacle of the soul or spirit? Are we to nourish it and treat it respectfully? Is it, instead, something intrinsically wicked, whose urges are to be suppressed at all costs? Or is the body something that is both to be valued and to be tamed? Do you think that it is in any way important to be concerned about the functioning and health of your body? Why?
- What does your tradition teach about the implications of destructive personal behavior, such as smoking, alcohol abuse, and overeating? Is it a sin? Is it to be avoided because

of its danger to the health of the body? Does it not really matter in the end, provided you are steadfast in your religious beliefs? Do you believe that God or a higher power cares whether or not you act in ways that are healthy?

- Do you follow the dos and don'ts of your religion or spiritual path when it comes to healthy behavior? Have you always done so, or have you recently been making more of an effort to do so? Have you noticed any changes in your health? What about in your mood or attitude toward life? Do you believe that there are spiritual benefits to living in accord with the teachings that you most value?

2

Religious Fellowship and Spiritual Support

Donna was fourteen years old and lived with her grandmother in a small town in Mississippi. For several years, Donna had been getting into more and more trouble, breaking the law and smoking marijuana, and skipping out on school. Then she became pregnant. Her grandmother was a prayerful woman, but realized that with a baby coming, Donna would soon be more than she could handle. Donna was sent to live with her aunt and uncle and cousins in Jackson.

Donna's relatives were members of the African Methodist Episcopal Church. Her uncle was a building contractor, her aunt was a nurse who helped run a church program that screened at-risk members for high blood pressure and diabetes once a month, and her three cousins were active in youth groups. One of them sang in the choir. From the day Donna moved in, it was made quite clear that she would attend church and take part in church activities. She was annoyed at first, but her aunt and uncle never left any room for doubt that they loved her unconditionally, and never once spoke a word in judgment of her pregnancy or other troubles.

A funny thing happened. Donna spent so much time in church—twice a week, typically—and felt so much pressure to do her homework and complete her chores, that she stopped getting into trouble. She did not have the time. Plus, with her baby due after the end of the school year, she had to start taking better care of herself. Her aunt made sure of that.

Right before her baby was born, Donna began to notice a change in her heart as well. She realized that she soon would have responsibility for another life, and this encouraged her to take more responsibility for herself and to think about her future. She also started enjoying church, and often went of her own accord to take part in after-school church activities. One Sunday morning during services, she accepted Jesus as her Lord and Savior.

By the time she got her diploma three years later, Donna had matured into a responsible young mother. She planned to go to the local community college and study to become a nurse, just like her aunt. Donna would tell anyone who asked that she owed everything to the love she had received from her family and from Christ and her church.

Going to church had benefited Donna's life in tangible ways as well. She had made many wonderful friends through her congregation, and the fellowship she shared with them made her feel accepted. Every other week, she and some of her friends would get together for Bible study with the assistant minister. If she needed to take her baby to the doctor and her aunt was at work, one of them or one of the church ladies would drive her. She also took part in a well-baby program at church, both as a client and a volunteer, and gave her time to another church program by talking to other teenagers about drugs and alcohol.

Donna especially loved the pastor's weekly sermons. She would always leave church inspired. The pastor was a wonderful man who had been over for dinner at her aunt and uncle's house many times. He always had the same message for Donna. He taught her that God cared about what happened to her and her baby and had a plan for their lives. He never ceased to remind her that there was something uniquely special for the Kingdom of God that only Donna and her baby could contribute. Every time he told her that, Donna would become so overcome by emotion that she could barely get out a "thank you."

Today Donna is in her late twenties. She is married and has two more children. She and her husband moved to Georgia, where she works part-time as a nurse. Donna volunteers for a church-based screening program that she co-founded, much like the one her aunt worked at in Mississippi. Neither she nor her husband uses cigarettes or alcohol, and their children are being raised in the church. She laughs sometimes when she thinks that she has become just as clean-living and wholesome as the nice church ladies she remembers as a teenager. She imagines that if her fourteen-year-old self could meet her current self, she would think she had gone crazy. That image always makes her smile.

Most Americans affiliate themselves with a religion or religious denomination and many agree, at least in principle, with the beliefs espoused by their particular faith tradition. As we saw in the last chapter, religious affiliation has a definite impact on health. When we identify with a particular faith or become a member of a religious institution, we are exposed to positive health-related messages and to a community of believers who may encourage us in our efforts to live by the tenets of our faith. In this way, religious affiliation can influence us to engage in healthy behaviors and lifestyle practices that reduce our risk of illness and promote greater health and well-being.

But just saying we belong to a religious group is not the same as actually being involved in religion. While most Americans report a religious affiliation, fewer actually participate in organized religious activities such as regularly attending worship services at church or synagogue. National surveys consistently report that just over 40 percent of adults attend religious services at least weekly. These numbers have not changed much for decades, and may be declining somewhat. Recent evidence suggests that this level of attendance may even be exaggerated to no small extent. One authoritative study compared people's reports of religious attendance in national surveys with actual counts of people attending a representative sample of Protestant and Catholic churches. The researchers concluded that real levels of weekly attendance are approximately one-half of those reported in surveys.

Whether 40 percent or 20 percent or some proportion in between, far fewer adult Americans are frequent participants in organized religious activities than are affiliated with a religion. Does regular involvement with church or synagogue, or other organized spiritual pursuits, have additional health implications above and beyond the beneficial effects of religious affiliation? The answer is a resounding yes.

Dozens of published studies have revealed numerous positive effects that frequent attendance at religious services consistently has on health. The salutary effect of regular religious attendance is even more striking than the link between religious affiliation and lower rates of illness. Like the data on affiliation reviewed in the previous chapter, studies of regular participation represent a largely unpublicized treasure trove of information, unfamiliar to most physicians and medical scientists. Until recently, these findings were not taught to medical students or residents, and have not been the stuff of continuing medical education or medical board exams. But the effect is as consistent and persuasive as for any important epidemiologic variable.

Is Frequent Religious Attendance Conducive to Better Health?

Back in my days as a graduate student at the University of Texas Medical Branch in the mid-1980s, my research on religious factors in health began to attract the attention of the hospital chaplains. A blurb in the campus newspaper about one of my studies caught the eye of the person in charge of the chaplains' biweekly noon seminar series. I was invited to address an audience of mostly ministers, priests, and nuns. The talk went well, but more significantly, I had the good fortune to meet someone with whom I would collaborate frequently over the next several years. Dr. Harold Y. Vanderpool, Harvard-trained bioethicist, medical historian, religious scholar, and professor of medical humanities, having no other lunch plans that day, decided to walk over to hear my presentation, which he saw advertised in a medical school flyer.

After my talk, Dr. Vanderpool introduced himself, and we hit it off immediately. I made an appointment to visit him in his office, and so began a relationship that was responsible, among other things, for the theoretical model of how religion relates to health that is the basis for this book. He informed me that while religion may be an obscure topic of research within the field of medicine, within the field of religious studies there has been a long-standing tradition of scholarly writing on health and medicine. Dr. Vanderpool, it turned out, was one of the premier authorities in the world.

I told Dr. Vanderpool of my efforts at the time to track down all of the published studies of religious differences in rates of morbidity and mortality. He was especially interested when I mentioned that along the way, I had also found more than two dozen studies that had examined how the frequency of attendance at religious services affected health. He believed that this material merited its own summary, and we quickly decided to write a detailed review article on the topic. It is one thing, he noted, to report that rates of health and illness vary across religious denominations. It would be quite another to provide evidence that regular attendance at services—a marker of actually *practicing* and not just professing religion—is beneficial for health.

By the time we completed our review, we had found a total of twenty-seven studies that examined the health effects of the frequency of attendance at religious services. Of these studies, twenty-two reported a statistically significant, positive association between religious attendance and health. That is, the more frequently one attended religious services, the lower the rate of whatever disease was being studied, or the higher the self-rating of health. These results were electrifying; we had no idea they would be so consistent.

The positive link between religious attendance and health persisted regardless of the particular illness or health condition examined in different studies. This mirrored the pattern that we found when examining the health effects of religious affiliation. We identified studies reporting beneficial effects of frequent attendance on all sorts of health and illness measures: atherosclerotic and degenerative heart disease deaths, cervical cancer incidence, cardiovascular pattern, depression, hypertension, neonatal mortality, Pap smear results, self-rated health, suicide symptoms, total mortality, trichomoniasis prevalence, and tuberculosis case rate.

The Epidemiology of Religion

Along with the write-up of what we found, we included a critique of the methodology of these studies, and Dr. Vanderpool added a lucid "brief primer on religion for epidemiologists." We entitled our paper "Is Frequent Religious Attendance *Really* Conducive to Better Health?" Somewhere in the final editing process, we conjured up the phrase "epidemiology of religion." Emboldened, we submitted the paper to a leading epidemiology journal. The paper was peer-reviewed and received both positive and negative feedback.

The editor's cover letter to us went on for nearly two single-spaced pages, specifying in painstaking detail how unacceptable, even misguided, our paper was, and urging us to give up the idea altogether and not pursue it any further. Unless you are a scientist, it is hard to comprehend how downright bizarre it was to receive such a letter from the editor of a peer-reviewed scientific journal. Most rejection letters contain a couple of paragraphs of boilerplate, signed by the editor or by his or her secretary, usually but not always including reviewers' comments. For this editor to take the time to go on and on about a paper that he was not even inviting to be revised and resubmitted, and to be somewhat unfriendly about it, seemed unprecedented. But that was not all. In his letter, he made sure to let us know that not only was our paper unacceptable, but the very *idea* of an epidemiology of religion was, in his words, "execrable."

I had to look the word up in a dictionary. For several years after, I believed it derived from the same root as "excretion" or "excrement," and concluded that the editor was telling us that not only our work, but our very ideas, were full of you-know-what. A few years later, as I related this story to a group of chaplains at the local Veterans Administration hospital, one of them, a Catholic priest and Latin expert, assured me that the word derived not from excretion but "execration." Before I could grab a dictionary, he told me that it meant "worthy of being detested, abominated, or abhorred." "Ah, that's a whole lot better," I said, and we all laughed.

Soon after we received our "execrable" review, our paper was published in *Social Science and Medicine*. This outstanding British journal has had the great foresight to publish many of the important studies in this field. Such open-mindedness to new ideas, sad to say, is uncharacteristic of many U.S. medical journals.

Health Benefits of Church Attendance

What was it about our review that had so upset the editor of the journal where we first submitted our paper? Maybe it was findings such as these:

1. Using data on Mexican Americans collected by my mentor, Dr. Kyriakos S. Markides of the University of Texas Medical Branch, we found that frequent church attenders were more likely to rate their health as good or excellent, report higher levels of well-being, and experience less disability, fewer days in bed in the previous year, and fewer physical symptoms.

2. A Scottish study found that active churchgoers, regardless of religious affiliation, had fewer physical and mental symptoms than people who affiliated with a religion but did not participate in church. These included members of the Church of Scotland, other types of Protestants, Roman Catholics, and non-Christians. But what religion one belonged to did not matter—only whether one actively participated in church.

3. Scientists from the University of Michigan, using data from the Tecumseh Community Health Study, found protective effects for frequent church attendance on heart disease in both sexes, and on mortality in women. Church attendance more than once a week offered an additional *31 percent reduction* in risk above and beyond weekly attendance.

4. Scientists at Johns Hopkins University, using data from an epidemiologic census of more than 90,000 people, found that less than monthly religious attendance *doubled and even tripled* the risk of death due to arteriosclerotic heart disease, pulmonary emphysema, cirrhosis of the liver, suicide, and cancers of the rectum and colon.

5. A follow-up study found an actual *dose-response* relationship between total deaths and frequency of religious attendance. Among people who never attended church, the annual death rate per 100,000 was 2,591.3. For those who attended church less than twice a year, it was 1,640.1; for those attending two to twelve times a year, 1,511.7; once a month, 1,354.3; and once a week or more, 1,308.1. Each level of frequency reduced deaths incrementally; attending services at least weekly reduced by *almost 50 percent* the risk of death the following year.

Take it from an epidemiologist—these last results are uncanny. They are more like something you would find in data on the relationship between cigarette smoking and the development of lung cancer. But there is more. Health benefits result not just from attendance at formal religious services, but from participation in other types of church activities. A study of churchgoers in Evans County, Georgia, for example, found that active participation in church groups led to lower rates of overall mortality. This interesting finding did not depend upon age, sex, or ethnicity. A protective effect was found in those under sixty years of age and those sixty years of age or older, in Caucasian men and women, and in African American women.

Don't Ask, Don't Tell

To be honest, Dr. Vanderpool and I did not mind that our call for an epidemiology of religion was considered "execrable." We figured that we must have hit a nerve. After all, for a scientist, the one thing worse than being despised or derided is being ignored.

But why the animosity? Epidemiologists, like any other species of scientist, do not appreciate being told that they have overlooked something vitally important that is right in front of their face. Perhaps our collation of so many positive findings unknown to so many in the field was in some way embarrassing. Perhaps scientists tend to be less religiously inclined than other folks, and do not wish to see faith placed in a positive light. Both of these may be true, but I think there is more to it than that.

Reflecting on why studying the health effects of religious participation should be considered unworthy of direct examination by epidemiologists, Dr. Vanderpool and I had noted that "epistemologically speaking, the domain and effects of religious commitment are believed to be unknowable or unreal or both. Western biomedicine, of which epidemiology is a part, is still wrestling with a body-mind dualism that defies consensus; thus, for most epidemiologists any resolution of a body-mind-spirit pluralism is simply beyond consideration."

In other words, "don't ask, don't tell." Some topics are simply taboo for scientists, and it seems that promising leads ought not to be followed if the results make too many people uncomfortable. Fortunately, many researchers have begun ignoring this advice. A large body of newly published findings sheds additional light on the relationship between organized religious participation and health.

New Findings from a National Study

In the years since our review article was published, many more studies have explored the health effects of organized religious participation. My research team colleagues and I began to take a special interest, and with the support of the National Institutes of Health (NIH), I initiated a program of systematic research on this topic. Along with Drs. Robert Joseph Taylor and Linda M. Chatters of the University of Michigan and Christopher G. Ellison of the University of Texas, and several other colleagues on occasion, I have published a series of research studies that document the effects of frequent religious attendance on a variety of indicators of health and overall well-being.

Using data from the approximately 2,000 people interviewed for the National Survey of Black Americans (NSBA), a nationally representative sample of African Americans in the United States, my colleagues and I examined the effects of a scale of "organizational religiosity." This scale summarized responses to questions on the frequency of attendance at religious services, official membership in a place of worship, participation in church clubs or organizations and other types of church activities, and serving as an officer at church.

Organized religious participation was a strong determinant of both health and psychological well-being. Moreover, the effect on well-being persisted *even after controlling for the effects of health*. This result was unexpected, and frankly shocking. Researchers had long presumed that health was the most important determinant of well-being; religion tended to be downplayed or simply ignored. This study confirmed that, on the contrary, active participation in church is more important than health. This finding flew in the face of conventional wisdom, and has caused a reconsideration of the influence of religion on well-being.

These results were published in the *Journal of Gerontology: Social Sciences*, the leading journal for studies of social factors in aging. When the NIH convened its first conference on the topic of religion and health in 1995, we were delighted to learn that our article was one of only three studies to receive a perfect "10," according to an NIH-commissioned rating of the scientific merit of all published studies in this field since 1975.

Replicating Our Results in Three National Studies

On the heels of this success, we decided to replicate these findings using data from several large, nationally representative studies conducted over a period of two decades. We wanted to see whether the effects that we had observed in African Americans extended to the overall population.

We obtained data on nearly 6,000 adults from the National Council on Aging's Myth and Reality of Aging study, and from the Quality of American Life and Americans' Changing Lives studies, both conducted at the University of Michigan. Each study assessed organized religious participation and aspects of health and well-being. This allowed us to examine the robustness of a religion-health association across study samples, time periods, and particular ways of assessing health. Research of this type, which looks at the relationship between a risk or protective factor and health in multiple studies, is known as "replicated secondary data analysis." If a specific finding is to merit our highest trust, it ought to be observable regardless of when or where a study was conducted and how the key variables were measured.

We observed significant effects from organized religious participation in all three study samples. These included strong salutary associations with how much of a problem health presents, overall health, satisfaction with health, activity limitation, presence of chronic diseases in the previous year, and dimensions of the well-known Affect Balance Scale. The results showed clearly that religious attendance exhibits beneficial effects according to a range of health indicators.

Health Effects Over Time

My colleagues and I also have explored this relationship longitudinally through what is known as "panel analysis." In a longitudinal study, multiple waves of data collection take place, separated by specific time intervals. When scientists can investigate changes that occur over time, we can more accurately chart the relationship between an exposure (e.g., religious attendance) and subsequent health. We can avoid the chicken-versus-egg speculation that often results from cross-sectional surveys.

Our most recent studies have verified that the benefits of religious attendance extend many years into the future—many, many years. My colleague Dr. Ellison examined data from the North Carolina sample of the NIH Epidemiologic Catchment Area (ECA) study. Nearly 3,000 people were surveyed in 1982–1983 and again a year later. More frequent religious attendance resulted in less depression, as measured by the authoritative Diagnostic Interview Schedule. Results controlled for the presence of chronic illnesses, stressful life conditions, and several sociodemographic factors known to influence mental health and well-being. This important study showed that frequent church attendance at a given point in time could help to prevent subsequent mood disorders *up to a year later*.

Religious attendance did even better in another study. Using data from more than 600 Mexican American adults in three generations, we investigated the effects of church attendance, assessed in 1981–1982, on well-being, assessed in 1992. Our most interesting finding involved the youngest generation (average age twenty-seven at baseline). The more frequently these young Mexican Americans attended church services, the less depression they had *eleven years later*.

The implications of these research findings are unmistakable. For the adults that we studied, how often one attends church has much to say about the extent to which one exhibits depressive symptoms up to a decade or more into the future. Psychiatrists know of few if any other factors that exhibit protective effects extending so far ahead in time. For sure, there is no medication that can work so effectively for so long.

The NSBA study's addition of a longitudinal component presented an opportunity to replicate our findings in a nationally representative sample of African Americans. As with our Mexican American study, we examined effects of baseline religious attendance on subsequent psychological well-being. In the NSBA, we had available to us measures of life satisfaction and happiness, as well as a version of the RAND Mental Health Index, a well-known validated scale assessing psychological distress. The original NSBA took place in 1979–1980, and subsequent waves of data were collected in 1987–1988, 1988–1989, and 1992.

We found that frequent church attendance exhibited a strong effect on life satisfaction and happiness assessed *twelve to thirteen years later*. Participation in other church activities also had comparable effects on both well-being measures. These findings outdid our results of an eleven-year protective effect among Mexican Americans. The principal investigators of the NSBA, located at the prestigious Institute for Social Research of the University of Michigan, have plans for a new round of data collection sometime after the year 2000. It will be interesting to see just how far the immunizationlike effects of frequent religious attendance actually extend.

If the results of several recent studies are any indication, our findings are not exceptional. We may even be considerably underestimating the scope and duration of the protective effect of going to religious services. This effect extends beyond health self-ratings and scales of emotional well-being. There is increasing evidence of religious effects on objective measures of more physically observable phenomena, such as functional disability and mortality. This effect also apparently extends decades into the future.

Two of the most prominent psychosocial epidemiologists in the world, Dr. Ellen L. Idler of Rutgers University and Dr. Stanislav V. Kasl of Yale, investigated the impact of religious attendance on physical functioning and disability. Using data on more than 900 older adults from the New Haven, Connecticut, sample of the multisite NIH Epidemiologic Study of the Elderly (EPESE), Drs. Idler and Kasl discovered that frequent attendance in 1982 was a strong determinant of better functioning through 1988, *six years later*, and a comparably strong but not quite statistically significant determinant through 1994, *twelve years later.*

The best study conducted to date on the topic of religious attendance and health also found the most amazing result. It showed that the protective effects of frequent participation in church can last a lifetime. Dr. William J. Strawbridge and colleagues at the Human Population Laboratory in Berkeley, California, examined data on more than 5,000 people from the famous Alameda County Study, with an eye to the possible protective effects of frequent religious attendance on subsequent mortality. Published in the *American Journal of Public Health*, their landmark study found that frequent religious attenders had greater survival rates—that is, lower mortality—that extended *over a twenty-eight-year period.* Frequent religious attendance in 1965 was still reducing the risk of dying in 1994. This study was impeccably done, controlling for baseline physical and mental health and health practices, and other factors known to be associated with religious attendance, mortality, or both. It did not matter. The preventive effect of religious attendance remained.

Links in a Chain:
Religious Participation→Social Support→Health

In exploring the experience of organized religious participation— what actually goes on when you attend church or synagogue—we can begin to find clues that help us make sense of all of these findings implicating religious attendance in preventing illness and death and promoting better health. We already have seen how the health benefits of religious affiliation are likely due to the effects of healthy behavior; now we can identify what the link is between religious attendance and health.

Religious attendance is a social behavior—it is not practiced in isolation. When we go to church or synagogue or to any other spiritual gathering, we take our place among fellow believers, for the most part—participants with us in a common activity. For sure, we may be present for different reasons: to praise God, to worship with others, to satisfy a spouse or parent, out of loneliness or boredom, to get a prayer answered, or to gain social acceptability. Regardless, studies tell us just being with other people, sharing a common purpose, is a well-known protective factor associated with decreased risk of illness and death and higher levels of health and well-being. Scientists call this factor "social support."

I believe that the supportive relationships provided through active religious fellowship best explain the findings we have examined. To demonstrate this, we first need to examine scientific evidence linking religious participation to social support, and social support to health. Both links are well established.

Social Support: What It Is and What It Does

For decades, sociologists and psychologists have explored the nuances of supportive relationships among people. Social support has come to be one of the principally invoked concepts in social science research of all types, especially in studies of health and well-being and responses to life stress. By now, thousands upon thousands of published studies have addressed conceptual, theoretical, and psychometric (measurement) issues in social support, or have provided empirical findings linking social support to a myriad of outcomes or predictors. "Social support" has almost become something of a buzzword in research circles. What exactly do scientists mean by the term?

Definitions abound, and the concept has been divided up in all sorts of ways. Researchers distinguish between the quantity and the quality of social contacts, emphasizing the structure and content of people's social networks and relationships. Similarly, a distinction is often made between availability and adequacy of support in disparate domains, from material assistance to intimate relationships. Others differentiate between perceived support—the thought or feeling that one is supported by or connected to other people—and enacted support—the helpful actions that are performed for the benefit of others.

A related distinction is often made between tangible and emotional support. Tangible support may consist of financial assistance, physical aid, or other forms of help and advice. A referral or a ride to a health care provider is a good example of tangible social support. Emotional support is sometimes referred to as an intangible form of social support. It may take the form of encouragement, guidance, or friendship. Whereas tangible social support is typically assessed through sociological measures of the giving and receiving of all kinds of social resources, emotional support has more to do with psychological or interpersonal transactions among people. It is more about the good feelings that pass from one to another—much like the Yiddish concept of *nachus*, extreme joy or pleasure.

Research over the past thirty to forty years has shown how social support, regardless of how it is defined or measured, can be a buffer against the harmful effects of stressful life changes. According to Dr. Peggy A. Thoits, this "buffering hypothesis," as it has come to be known, suggests that "individuals with a strong social support system should be better able to cope with major life changes; those with little or no social support may be more vulnerable to life changes, particularly undesirable ones."

Numerous studies strongly support this contention.

In his presidential address to the American Psychosomatic Society in 1976, Dr. Sidney Cobb reviewed evidence that social support moderated the effects of stress caused by a variety of problems across the life course. These included situations as diverse as pregnancy complications, hospitalization, recovery from tuberculosis, employment termination, retirement, and bereavement. The greater or more effective the social support, the less the frequency or severity of these problems. Dr. Cobb concluded, "We have seen strong and often quite hard evidence, repeated over a variety of transitions in the life cycle from birth to death, that social support is protective."

Religious Fellowship as a Form of Social Support

In his presidential address, Dr. Cobb defined social support as "information leading the subject to believe that he is cared for and loved, esteemed, and a member of a network of mutual obligations."

This sounds an awful lot like what goes on in formal religious institutions such as churches, synagogues, and groups organized for meditation or spiritual study—at least in principle. Research on the functional contributions of religion throughout the course of adult life indeed supports this connection between religious fellowship and the giving and receiving of social support. Much of this research comes from studies in gerontology—an interdisciplinary field that focuses on the aging process from early adulthood through the elderly years.

Dr. Christopher G. Ellison, my research colleague, has described how active religious participation benefits health and overall well-being. In his chapter in my book *Religion in Aging and Health*, he develops a model of the ways that religious involvement enables the receipt of social support.

1. Religious fellowship provides both tangible and emotional resources that buffer or reduce our experience of stress, whether it is caused by major life events, chronic stressors, or daily hassles. Formal involvement in religious communities reduces the likelihood of experiencing stressors such as chronic and acute illness, marital tension and dissolution, and work-related and legal problems. Sociological studies bear this out.

2. Active religious participation increases the likelihood that when stressful situations arise, they are put in a larger context that offers greater meaning, and therefore are experienced less negatively. In Dr. Ellison's words, religion provides "cognitive and institutional frameworks that make certain stressors seem less threatening to an individual than they might otherwise appear." These include psychological resources such as theological worldviews that make sense out of a chaotic world; favorable psychological states or traits; self-esteem and feelings of self-efficacy or personal mastery; and a sense of connection to a benevolent "divine other." Such in-

ner resources may alter our perceptions of stressful circumstances and strengthen our coping skills and ability to deal with stress, thereby reducing its potentially harmful impact.

3. Regular religious fellowship increases our access to people who can offer us assistance when we are in need. Frequent participants in worship services, for example, are plugged into a network of friends and family with whom they spend time on a regular basis, have gotten to know, and to whom and from whom they can give and receive both tangible and emotional support. This may include encouragement and good cheer, and the *nachus* mentioned earlier, as well as health advice or a ride to the doctor.

Research on Religion and Social Support

In theory, active religious participation can be a source of support, which in turn may help to buffer the effects of stress and promote well-being. Does scientific evidence back up these assertions? Dr. Ellison's own research has done much to confirm the ways in which active religious involvement helps to establish social ties and provide social support.

Along with sociologist Dr. Linda K. George of Duke University, a past president of the Gerontological Society of America, Dr. Ellison used data from the North Carolina ECA study to examine how frequent church attendance affected characteristics of social support. Frequent churchgoers enjoyed larger social networks of non–family members; had more contact with members of their social networks; received more varied types of social support, whether tangible (financial assistance, helping with errands, advice, transportation, helping with meals or illnesses) or emotional; and experienced more favorable perceptions of the quality of their social relationships. Frequent church attenders were also more likely to rate these relationships as favorable regardless of age, sex, ethnicity, or marital status.

Drs. Robert Joseph Taylor and Linda M. Chatters, the other members of our research team, have examined the effect of religious participation on receipt of informal types of support. By "informal support" they mean those types of assistance other than the formal social services often delivered to congregants by religious institutions. Over the years, using data from the NSBA study, they have identified many interesting links between religious involvement and social support among African Americans.

- More frequent church attendance is associated with receiving needed support more often and in greater amounts. Types of support included advice and encouragement, companionship, goods and services, financial assistance, transportation, help during sickness, and prayer.
- Among older adults, frequent church attendance increases the probability of receiving support. Frequent attenders are also less likely ever to need support. This jibes well with Dr. Ellison's assertion that religious participation both increases access to supportive resources and prevents circumstances whereby they are needed.
- Among the elderly, whereas two-thirds of people received support from their extended family, three-quarters received support from church members. Almost 60 percent of people received church support "fairly often" or "very often"; for family support, the comparable figure was one-third.

Supportive Relationships: The Secret to Health, Happiness, and Long Life?

In 1988, a most unusual article appeared in *Science*, the world's leading scientific journal. This essay, "Social Relationships and Health" by Drs. James S. House, Karl R. Landis, and Debra Umberson of the University of Michigan, summarized a quarter of a century of research on the importance of "social integration" for health. This they defined as the presence of a number of socially supportive relationships, such as with family and friends, also taking into account the structure of such relationships (i.e., their "density" and "reciprocity") and their actual content. The concept of social support long had been a principal focus of study among social epidemiologists, due in part to influential earlier work by Dr. Berton H. Kaplan and his colleagues, Drs. John C. Cassel and Susan Gore, of the University of North Carolina. The idea that low levels of social support might be a certifiable risk factor for illness, across the board, was less well known to physicians and to basic scientists in other fields.

Dr. House and his associates reviewed findings from many of the classic longitudinal studies in epidemiology. The roll call of these studies is familiar to any public health scientist: Evans County; Tecumseh; North Karelia, Finland; Alameda County. Their findings "manifest a consistent pattern of results," and House and associates wasted no time in getting to the point: "More socially isolated or less socially integrated individuals are less healthy, psychologically and physically, and more likely to die."

The latter finding is especially stunning. Analyses of both women and men, and African Americans and Caucasians, show that people who receive less social support have a greater probability of decreased longevity and premature death. How strong is this effect? "The evidence on social relationships is probably stronger, especially in terms of prospective studies, than the evidence which led to the certification of the Type A behavior pattern as a risk factor for coronary heart disease."

That is not all. The authors further state that the death risk associated with low levels of social support appears to exceed that attributed to cigarette smoking in the famous Surgeon General's report of 1964.

Adding to the impact of their article, they cited research findings that controlling for the effects of health and various biological and personality factors was unable to explain away this harmful effect of low social support. In other words, after taking into account the likelihood that a relationship between social support and mortality was observed only because it reflected effects of other known determinants of mortality that happened to be correlated with social support, the effect was still present. House and his coauthors concluded, "Social relationships have a predictive, arguably causal, association with health in their own right."

Lack of Social Support:
A Fundamental Cause of Disease

This theme has been taken up recently by others. Based on the conclusions of House and several other researchers, a provocative article by scientists from Columbia University and UCLA, published in a recent special issue of the *Journal of Health and Social Behavior*, asserted that certain social conditions, including lack of social support, are "fundamental causes of disease."

Establishing the link between social support and health has probably been the greatest contribution of the field of social epidemiology. This relationship has been replicated in both males and females, across all age groups, in different ethnic groups and nations, and for a variety of diseases across various stages in the natural history or course of illness. Social support has exhibited protective, preventive, therapeutic, or otherwise salutary effects on numerous outcomes, such as the onset of depression, recovery from heart disease and cancer, and self-ratings of overall health.

At the conclusion of their *Science* article, House, Landis, and Umberson reiterated an important point for their largely nonsociological audience: "The extent and quality of social relationships experienced by individuals is [sic] also a function of broader social forces."

These, they emphasized, include attendance at church, a theme that House had explored in a research study on social support, religion, and mortality several years earlier. The possibility that frequent attendance exhibits protective effects against illness because it fosters health-promoting support is a reasonable hypothesis in light of existing theory and research findings.

In an article published in the *Journal for the Scientific Study of Religion* with my colleague Dr. Markides, I noted that a "social support explanation appears to be the central, unspoken assumption of epidemiologists working with religion variables." Based on studies explored in subsequent chapters of this book, that assumption may be overstated. But for those studies that focus on participation in organized religious activities, such as church or synagogue attendance, an explanation based in part on social support appears sound.

Lessons to Consider

The evidence in this chapter gives rise to our second principle of theosomatic medicine:

PRINCIPLE 2

Regular religious fellowship benefits health by offering support that buffers the effects of stress and isolation.

What can we learn from scientific studies linking organized religious participation to better health through receipt of social support? What do these findings tell us about the value for health and well-being of regular fellowship with other people? How can we derive the personal benefits of regular religious participation in our lives?

Regularly attending church or synagogue or other spiritual gatherings can have tangible and emotional benefits far beyond the spiritual contentment one may expect. These secular benefits may even outweigh the religious ones in their impact on our quality of life. This is not to say that we should be diligent in our religious participation only for the social and interpersonal gains that might accrue. But we all need companions. Unless we have taken monastic or ascetic vows, we need others—to work with, to play with, to live with, to love, and to worship with. Actually, most monks and ascetics do, too.

Not all of us enjoy attending formal religious services in a large organized church or religious institution, at least on a regular basis. For some, such services are cold and impersonal, and it is hard to feel much of a spiritual connection with God or the divine or holy. It depends a lot on what religion or denomination one belongs to, where one attends, who the clergyperson or leader is, and how the services are structured. But there are other ways to connect with people in spiritually oriented settings.

Most congregations provide a number of ways to join with other members in regular fellowship. These include boards and committees, social groups, community action groups, youth groups, choirs, book clubs, and so on. The synagogue that my wife and I belong to has more than twenty standing committees, formal groups, and classes, according to the most recent directory. Certainly, not every member attends worship services nearly every week—only a small fraction do—but congregants have ample opportunity to participate in organized activities that involve communing with other members on a regular basis.

Outside of formal religious institutions, we can become involved in supportive relationships through prayer circles, meditation groups, and classes organized to study the spiritual teachings of a particular spiritual tradition. In some communities, there are many existing groups to choose from, sometimes outnumbering the churches and often with older roots than any local religious institution.

For example, in Virginia Beach, Virginia, where we lived for many years, the Association for Research and Enlightenment (ARE) sponsors a prayer group known as the Glad Helpers. The ARE is a research and educational organization associated with the work of the late "sleeping prophet," Edgar Cayce. The purpose of the Glad Helpers is to offer up healing prayers for those who request them. This group has been meeting regularly, once a week, since 1931. Some of the original members still attend. There are churches and synagogues that cannot come close to that record of providing consistent and continuing fellowship for its members.

Questions to Reflect On

At the start of this chapter, I told you about Donna. Like many youngsters, she was caught up in behavior she could not control that was harmful and threatening to her future. Through good fortune—some would call it grace—she was able to move to a healthier environment, one in which participation in church with a supportive family took center stage. This resulted in dramatic transformations in both her inner and outer life.

Like Michael, about whom I spoke in Chapter 1, Donna's story is inspiring, but really not out of the ordinary. Many of us see marked improvements in our quality of life as a result of regular religious fellowship. For newly religious people, gains associated with fellowship may be especially great. Joining with others of a shared spiritual outlook can fill a void in one's life in ways that more secular types of social activities are unable to do.

Some of us renew ties to the denomination or congregation of our childhood. This is an increasingly common trend among young couples who drifted away from organized religion soon after confirmation, *bar* or *bat mitzvah*, or graduation from religious school. The birth of one's own children is often a powerful motivation to return to the faith in which one was raised. Churches and synagogues are excellent sources of companionship and education for children, and help to establish a sense of tradition and continuity. For parents, there can be great satisfaction in reconnecting with old familiar friends, both human and institutional—liturgies, prayers, songs, holiday cycles, youth groups.

Others of us choose to convert to a new religion or spiritual path. Often this follows years of searching. Connecting with a new spiritual home means making new acquaintances and developing new relationships. As we establish new traditions, we integrate ourselves into support networks that may provide us with tangible or emotional resources to benefit our well-being. We also may be presented with opportunities to provide support to others.

I can relate to both examples. As a teenager, especially once I left for college, I drifted far from Jewish observance. I was what is called a "twice-a-year Jew": I attended synagogue for the High Holy Days each fall, and never failed to celebrate Passover and Chanukah, but little in my daily life reflected a commitment to Judaism. I began studying the spiritual traditions of the world, not just as a religious scholar but at times as a participant. The "inner," or mystical, path especially interested me. But I did not seek organized religious fellowship; I pursued these interests mostly alone. My spiritual questing was private, and sometimes lonely. Although I was fulfilled in deeply meaningful ways, I missed the opportunity to be a part of a community of believers.

Eventually my journey took me full circle. By my late twenties, my interest in the mystical experience led me to the inner path within my own tradition, known as *kabbalah*. Through connections with the Jewish Renewal movement, I found myself back in synagogue regularly for the first time since I was a child. Today my wife and I are active members of our congregation. We worship with others at weekly *Shabbat* services, and I take part in several other group activities. These include the synagogue board, our social action committee, and regular Talmud study. We also have participated in a meditation group that includes a mix of synagogue members and friends from the community. These activities are a profound source of spiritual nourishment for me. The opportunity to get together to "do" and "be" in a spiritual way with others contributes to my mental health and well-being in ways that private devotion cannot match.

If you are involved in regular religious fellowship or if you actively participate in organized spiritual activities, then you have your own history and your own story to tell. For many people, getting together with others for spiritual pursuits is a source of great contentment, emotional nourishment, and growth. There are things that we can learn about ourselves and about God or the eternal only in the presence of other people. The powerful bonds that we form with fellow participants can benefit us in tangible ways as well, and just being around friends and acquaintances regularly is good for us in and of itself. Several questions can help us to reflect on how our formal religious and spiritual activities provide social benefits that affect our overall well-being.

1. What types of religious activities do you participate in at your place of worship? Do you attend services regularly, teach religious school, or volunteer for committees? Outside of your church or synagogue, or if you are not a member of one, do you ever get together with other people for spiritually oriented activities? Examples might include meditation groups, yoga classes, home- or work-based study or discussion or prayer groups.
2. Has your involvement in organized religious or spiritual activities led you to make new friends? Has it expanded your social circle? Are these friends and acquaintances sources of help and advice? Are you satisfied with the quality of these relationships?

Do you give as much as you receive when it comes to tangible and emotional support?

3. Do you believe that your involvement in spiritual group activities has had an effect on your emotional well-being? If you are a newly active participant, are you happier and more satisfied now that you have gotten involved? If you are a long-standing church- or synagogue-goer or participant in noncongregational activities, how does this fellowship affect the quality of your life? Do you look forward to religious services or group meetings? Would you get up out of a sickbed to attend, if you could? When you are unable to attend services, do you feel that you can still be there in spirit? When you are involved with others in spiritual activities, how does it make you feel? More alive? Stronger? Healthier? More connected to all people? Closer to God?

PART 2

The Health Effects of Private Spirituality

Public participation in organized activities is not the only way that people express themselves religiously. Private expressions of spirituality are a central and salient feature in the lives of many people whether or not they would describe themselves as formally religious. Part 2 explores the health benefits of private spiritual expression, emphasizing the psychological functions of spirituality. Through engendering wholesome and salutary emotions, beliefs, and thoughts, this private dimension of spirituality alleviates physical and psychological distress and promotes good health.

The chapters in Part 2 provide evidence supporting our next three principles of theosomatic medicine:

PRINCIPLE 3

Participation in worship and prayer benefits health through the physiological effects of positive emotions.

PRINCIPLE 4

Religious beliefs benefit health by their similarity to health-promoting beliefs and personality styles.

PRINCIPLE 5

Simple faith benefits health by leading to thoughts of hope, optimism, and positive expectation.

3

The Emotional Impact of Worship

Ruth loved her synagogue. A grandmother of three, she was an active member of the same congregation that she had belonged to most of her life. For so many years, every time there was an event at temple—a Shabbat *service, a special celebration for the children, a committee meeting—Ruth would be there. Besides her family, of course, her Jewish faith and her love of Torah and temple were the center of her life.*

Ruth especially looked forward to worship services. She loved the peace, the stillness as she sat holding her siddur, *praying with others and experiencing the presence of God. Worship gave her a sense of calm and contentment, and a relaxed feeling of wholeness.*

As Ruth got on in years, she began having health problems. Most were self-limiting—they would come and go—and none of them kept her away from temple for too long. Over time, though, her health problems became more serious, and they began to interfere with her synagogue activities. She started to have some rheumatological symptoms that made it increasingly difficult to get around. This condition made it painful to hold or carry things or be on her feet for long periods of time. Still, she persevered in her temple activities.

One day Ruth felt an intense pain. Her doctor checked her out and sent her for a lengthy series of tests. The doctor was honest with her; it might be cancer. There would be many more tests, and they would prove to be tiring, painful, and nerve-racking. Ruth was terrified, and for a while was too exhausted even to go to temple.

During the time she spent at home, Ruth began reading books on the role of feelings and emotions in promoting health and hastening recovery from illness.

She truly believed that a positive outlook was important, but it was hard to stay upbeat. Her preexisting conditions were difficult enough without having to deal with the threat of cancer. And without temple, she felt especially cut off from a source of deep joy. She became sad and depressed.

Fortunately, the tests came back negative; Ruth did not have cancer. Soon she was able to return to temple and take part in worship and other activities once more. Remembering what she had read, Ruth tried to be especially aware of her body and her feelings while at worship. Her sadness lifted, and that old feeling of calm and peace returned. She now has found that she can maintain these feelings even after services. All she has to do is close her eyes and silently pray, imagining herself sitting in temple, and she is flooded once more with a warm relaxation. For a moment, her heart beats slower, her joints and muscles ache less, her tension fades away, and she rejoices in the knowledge that she has heeded the biblical call to "be still and know that I am God" (Psalms 46:10).

"Consider your soul," suggested *Reader's Digest* in its article "Eight Easy Ways to Look—and Feel—Years Younger." Citing my work as evidence, the article named frequent churchgoing as the final key to "help you stay healthy, look and feel younger and live longer." Yet just as reporting a religious affiliation does not guarantee active religious participation, neither does frequent religious attendance necessarily imply anything more than sitting passively in a pew. As the previous chapter indicates, there is strong evidence from numerous studies that going to church or synagogue is associated with positive health outcomes, and we have a good idea why; but these studies do not tell us what goes on inside people's hearts once they walk through the door.

Not all people who attend services do so to worship collectively, to connect with God or a higher power, or to receive spiritual sustenance. For some, attendance is motivated by a desire to please their family; for others, a perceived need to appear socially acceptable; for still others, loneliness or boredom. For these people, the social support benefits of attendance may still be present. That is, even if active religious participation is motivated by reasons other than making some kind of connection with God or the divine, there are still considerable gains to be derived from fellowship with others.

But for people whose churchgoing or synagogue experience is motivated by a desire to experience the joy of worship, practicing religion may offer health benefits beyond those resulting from the effects of healthy habits and supportive networks. The worship experience may produce feelings such as hope, forgiveness, catharsis, and love, which science tells us can affect our physiology, promoting health and relieving distress. Just as research studies report benefits of religious affiliation and organized religious participation, so is there solid evidence that worshiping God has a positive influence on our health.

The Demography of Prayer

Research confirms that prayer is the most common form of worship. Among adult Americans, rates of prayer, both collectively and privately, have been uniformly high for decades.

Data from the authoritative General Social Survey reveal that over half of us pray at least daily, a trend that has held steady for nearly thirty years. Data from various surveys show that the proportion of us who report ever praying to God has held consistently at around 90 percent for over fifty years. If anything, levels of very frequent prayer seem to have increased. Sociologist Dr. Andrew M. Greeley notes that the number of people who reported praying more than once a day—certainly a good indicator of an active devotional life—rose from about a quarter of the population in the early to mid-1970s to nearly one-third a decade later.

Using a nationally representative sample of nearly 1,500 adults, my colleague Dr. Taylor and I explored in considerable depth the patterns of prayer among Americans. We analyzed data from the annual General Social Survey, the same source used by Dr. Greeley, to update and expand on his findings. We made several important observations:

1. Counting both public and private prayer, considerably more people pray at least daily than attend weekly religious services.

This includes over 43 percent of those ages eighteen to thirty, over 45 percent of those ages thirty-one to forty, over 57 percent of those ages forty-one to sixty, and nearly three-quarters of those over age sixty.

2. Hardly anyone reports that they never pray. Less than 1 percent of respondents said that they never engaged in prayer. This is consistent with other studies that have found this number to vary between 2 percent at the highest, and zero.

3. Prayer is more frequently practiced in successively older age groups. This could reflect higher rates of prayer in earlier generations, or it could mean that we pray more as we get older. Or it could mean both.

4. Women pray more often than men, throughout life, and African Americans pray more often than Caucasians.

5. The strongest determinant of frequent prayer is active participation in religious services.

Naturally, folks who go to church or synagogue regularly will have more opportunities, on average, to pray than those who do not. But many of us pray privately, for reasons unrelated to participation in formal worship liturgies. Other strong determinants of frequent prayer in our study were a feeling of closeness to God and a history of mystical or transcendent experiences.

Prayer is a natural part of most of our lives. It is a component of organized religious worship across religions and religious denominations, and also reflects and is motivated by very personal feelings and experiences. Prayer, whether public or private, is often used for "expressive" purposes—a term used by social scientists to mean "for its own sake." But it may also be used "instrumentally"—as a means to an end.

Do Religious Worship and Prayer Influence Health?

According to a study by my colleagues, Drs. Christopher G. Ellison and Robert Joseph Taylor, people also turn to prayer to deal with personal crises and issues. They do so for many reasons. Some of us pray out of a need for help with such personal problems as finances, the law, or conflicts with others. Others pray as a way to cope with bereavement. Others pray to seek healing. The use of prayer for purposes of coping depends upon the availability and closeness of others to pray with us or for us.

Regardless of whether prayer is used expressively or instrumentally, the consequences of an active prayer life for health and well-being are clear. Frequent prayer, whether public or private, is associated with better health and emotional well-being and lower levels of psychological distress. My colleagues and I have observed this relationship irrespective of ethnic group or religious denomination in a variety of longitudinal studies.

- Participants in a study of more than 500 older Mexican Americans and Anglo Caucasians, predominantly Catholics, were asked how often they prayed when not in church. Frequent private prayer strongly influenced well-being. The more often folks prayed, the greater their well-being *over eight years later*.
- We replicated these findings in over 2,000 adult African Americans, mostly Baptists and Methodists. Once again, there was a longitudinal effect: frequent prayer led to greater life satisfaction and happiness *over a decade later*.
- My colleague Dr. Ellison, along with his associates, investigated the effect of religious devotion in a nationally representative sample. Religious devotion was assessed by combining data on the frequency of prayer and feelings of connection to God. The intensity of devotion was a strong determinant of life satisfaction, regardless of one's level of religious attendance, religious affiliation, social interaction with others, health, or experience of traumatic life events in the past year.

This is a startling and important finding, and there is more here than meets the eye. According to these results, the benefit of religious devotion for well-being extends above and beyond any benefit attributable to religious affiliation or organized religious participation. Further, this benefit does not simply reflect the known health advantages of social support, nor does it disappear in the presence of traumatic life stress.

Replicating the Prayer-Health Connection at Duke

Other well-regarded scientists have confirmed that regular worship and prayer exhibit beneficial effects on health and well-being. Research conducted at Duke University has replicated a prayer-health connection in a variety of populations, age groups, ethnicities, and religious denominations.

A provocative study examined effects of religious devotion in more than 4,000 adult participants in the North Carolina EPESE study. Religious devotion was assessed by frequency of private religious activities such as prayer, meditation, and Bible study. The investigator, sociologist Dr. Marc A. Musick, was a graduate student at Duke at the time. He is now at the University of Texas, and is both a former student and current colleague of Dr. Ellison. Dr. Musick's results are quite interesting. He found that the more frequently people participated in devotional activities, the healthier they rated themselves. This held after controlling for other aspects of religiousness, key personal characteristics (age, sex, marital status), both healthy behavior and satisfactory social ties, and even objective measures of health such as previously diagnosed chronic diseases and functional impairment.

This landmark study is important for two reasons. First, it identifies an effect of religious devotion on what researchers term "subjective health." This is typically assessed by a single question (e.g., "In general, how would you rate your health: excellent, good, fair, or poor?"), which is commonly asked in epidemiologic studies. Subjective health is considered a reliable indicator of one's overall state of health, and one of the best predictors that we know of for mental health, level of functional disability, rates of physician use, and even longevity. Establishing a connection between religious worship and this key indicator is a sign that worship has very real consequences for our health.

Second, and more important, Dr. Musick's results demonstrate the robustness of a prayer-health connection. As with Dr. Ellison's findings for religious devotion and well-being described above, we now know that private devotion influences health *above and beyond* the benefits attributable to other dimensions of religious involvement and to practicing healthy behavior or receiving social support. However it is that religious worship impacts our health for the better, these findings tell us that it apparently does so in ways that religious affiliation and organized religious participation alone cannot.

Another notable Duke study explored the impact of prayer and religious devotion among older adults, a group well known to sociologists of religion for their more frequent private religious activities. Results were similar to Dr. Musick's, and showed that religious worship has implications for the well-being of the elderly as well as for younger adults.

This study of 1,100 people from Illinois drew on five groups of older adults: geriatric outpatients, participants in a state-sponsored seniors' lunch program, members of several conservative Protestant churches, participants in a Jewish seniors' lunch program, and retired Dominican and Franciscan nuns. The main study factor, "nonorganizational religious activity," was measured by combining data on several activities such as private prayer and devotional reading. Researchers, led by Dr. Harold G. Koenig, a geriatric psychiatrist at Duke University and the world's preeminent clinical scientist in the area of religion and health, found that frequent worship was associated with higher morale; less agitation, loneliness, and dissatisfaction with life; and greater ability to cope with tension. This was found overall, as well as in women, younger folks, older folks, sick folks, and healthy folks, regardless of religious affiliation.

Drs. Musick and Koenig have since joined forces for a longitudinal study of the effects of religious devotion on mental health. Using data from the North Carolina EPESE study, a composite measure of prayer, meditation, and Bible study was analyzed in relation to four dimensions of the well-regarded Center for Epidemiologic Studies Depression scale: depressive symptoms, positive affect (a happy mood), somatic-retarded activity (low energy, poor appetite), and poor interpersonal relations. The investigators were interested in whether religious devotion, assessed in 1986, would have any effect on the mental health of cancer patients in 1989. Among African Americans, effects of devotion on depressive symptoms, somatic-retarded activity, and poor interpersonal relations were as anticipated—suggesting a protective effect—but of insufficient magnitude to attain statistical significance. A significant effect was found, however, on emotions. Among African American cancer patients, frequent prayer, meditation, or Bible study led to a happy and contented mood *three years later, despite experiencing cancer.*

Links in a Chain:
Religious Worship→Positive Emotions→Health

We once again need to identify the "active ingredient" that connects religious worship to health. We must identify a factor that, like the link in a chain, is both an outcome of religious worship and a determinant of health. In Chapter 1, we observed how religious affiliation sanctions and reinforces healthy behaviors that protect against disease and death. In Chapter 2, we saw how organized religious participation provides social support that lessens the disease-making impact of life stress. What do we know about prayer and devotion that suggests how they might influence health?

I propose that the health benefits of worship and prayer are due to the health-promoting effects of the positive emotions that they engender. Religious worship produces and is characterized by distinct emotions, regardless of what spiritual path one follows. These run the gamut from healthy feelings ideally sought through devotion—peace, joy, trust, love—to destructive feelings sometimes unexpectedly encountered along the way—guilt, fear, anger, hatred. Regardless of the polarity of our feelings, positive or negative, scientific studies tell us that our emotions have a lot to say about our health.

From cutting-edge research in new fields such as psychophysiology and psychoneuroimmunology, we have learned that emotions are "hardwired" into our autonomic nervous, endocrine, and immune systems. As a consequence, what we feel can affect the physiological functioning of our bodies. Whatever affects what and how we feel therefore has a clear path, physiologically speaking, to influence our body and our mind. Whatever elicits heartfelt emotional responses is a potentially protective factor, epidemiologically speaking, and deserves our scrutiny. In this regard, religious worship has few equivalents.

Religious Worship and Emotional Attachments

Dr. Susan H. McFadden and I recently described how religious worship works to influence the feelings that we experience in our daily lives. Dr. McFadden, a psychologist at the University of Wisconsin at Oshkosh, is one of the preeminent figures in the field of religious gerontology. She was selected to write the chapter on religion and spirituality in the *Encyclopedia of Gerontology*, a sign of her considerable stature in this field.

In our chapter in the *Handbook of Emotion, Adult Development, and Aging*, we presented a perspective on the interconnections among religion, emotions, and health. At best, worshiping publicly with others elicits feelings of interpersonal trust, mutuality, and intimacy. Group rituals, such as prayer, give structure and context to our encounters with God or the divine. Worship activates what psychologists call "attachment" processes that connect people both to one another and to their conception of a spiritual force or to God. Holding to an image of God as a loving heavenly father, as in Judaism, Christianity, and Islam, or as a divine mother, as in neopaganism and some New Age spiritual paths, is an example of a loving attachment nurtured by worshiping with others.

Private observance, too, may reinforce similar emotional attachments. Through home-based prayer, daily devotions, and meditation, feelings may be produced that serve to connect us with fellow believers, now and throughout history, and with God or one's "higher self." For older adults especially, worship experiences emphasize the intrinsic and enduring meaning of life, fostering a sense of feeling blessed by God. This may be vital for elderly people struggling to "preserve the self" in the face of circumstances that may prevent them from maintaining their lifelong patterns of worship in church or synagogue.

How and Why We Pray

Not all worship is the same. According to Dr. Margaret M. Poloma, a sociologist and professor at the University of Akron and one of the world's foremost experts on how and why people pray, prayer can be divided into four categories. Ritual prayer includes reading from prayer books or reciting memorized prayers, like those found in the Jewish *siddur* or Catholic missal. Conversational or colloquial prayer is characterized as informally talking with God. Petitionary prayer requests that spiritual or material needs be filled by God or the universe. Meditative prayer entails thinking about God or the divine, listening for God's voice, or in the words of sixteenth-century Carmelite monk Brother Lawrence, "practicing the presence of God."

To quote one of my papers: "These types of prayer are not mutually exclusive; for instance, many individuals who utilize ritual prayer also engage in more informal conversational prayer. If there is a sine qua non to these disparate styles of prayer, it may be, as James long ago noted, the seeking of an 'inward communion' with the divine, leading the pray-er 'into the presence of the ultimate mystery of God.'"

Prayer and worship are means to connect us to God or the eternal, whether directly, as some religions believe, or through participation in a fellowship of believers. Among observant Jews, for example, certain prayers are recited at prescribed times daily (the *shema, birkhat hamazon*), weekly (the *berakhah* for the *Shabbat* candles), monthly (*rosh chodesh*), and yearly (at Yom Kippur), or as circumstances arise (*yizkor, mi shebayrach, shehecheyanu*). Some of these prayers are a part of public worship liturgies conducted in a *minyan* at *shul;* others are privately recited at home, alone or with one's family. In both cases, these prayers connect the pray-er to all others throughout the world who are praying the same thing at the same time. Prayer is therefore a powerful means to enhance one's feelings of connection to others "horizontally," extending bonds of solidarity across a community of believers; "vertically," linking those who pray to God; and throughout time, forging bridges to fellow worshipers across history.

In *How I Pray*, journalist Jim Castelli interviewed over two dozen people from many of the world's faith traditions. Their stories are testament to the power of prayer to evoke emotions that connect us to God through connecting us to fellow worshipers. One interviewee, a Jewish woman, described how her prayer life had changed as she grew and matured. As a teenager, she had participated in a Reform Jewish youth group that experimented with unstructured and contemporized prayers mixing liturgy with poetry or creative reading. As an adult, she found that this was no longer enough for her.

> I've since grown out of that type of prayer—although I still see its importance for the high school students with whom I work. I used to pray that way, but during my college career I learned more Hebrew and became comfortable praying in an Orthodox atmosphere where it was all Hebrew. I was drawn to the traditional Jewish prayers because I like the feeling that the words I'm saying out of the prayer book are words that Jews all around the world are saying. There is time for personal prayer in the liturgy, but I've become very connected to the idea of the tradition that goes on, and that is that all Jews on Friday evenings are saying the same thing, with their own personal additions.

Worship, Prayer, and Mood

According to the late Dr. Joachim Wach, University of Chicago historian of religions, worship works "to bind together and unite those animated by the same central experience." Besides formal or informal prayer, other worship experiences—"cultic acts," in the language of religious scholars—also strongly influence our moods and attitudes and thus work to integrate people. These essential functions of religion include festivals, pilgrimages, purifications, lustrations, vows, offerings, sacrifices, and processions. Participation in such acts of worship can produce commonly experienced emotional responses among fellow believers that reinforce their mutual ties.

The nineteenth-century philosopher and psychologist Dr. William James, in his classic *The Varieties of Religious Experience*, explained that expressions of religiousness may reflect or contribute to two types of religious feelings. People who adhere to "healthy-minded" religion experience the world as good, feel harmoniously connected to all things, and gain immediate happiness through their spiritual life. By contrast, the religion of "sick souls" leads them to see the world as sinful and evil, to feel mostly guilt and fear, and to derive sadness and melancholy from the practice of their faith. James saw some value in these "morbid-minded" emotions. At least such responses were not blind to the evil that exists in the world. Healthy-minded religion, in its extreme form, is a faith of rose-colored glasses. The most balanced type of religiousness, for James, would be neither overly optimistic nor overly pessimistic. It would see reality as it is; worshipers, in turn, would experience neither extreme highs nor extreme lows.

Salutary Emotions: The Case of Norman Cousins

In 1964, Norman Cousins, well-known editor of *The Saturday Review*, was overcome by a crippling illness that landed him in the hospital in a state of constant pain. Cousins, an avid reader of scientific and medical literature, suspected that he was suffering from adrenal exhaustion and a general dysfunction or shutdown of his endocrine system. As he wondered what he would do next, a thought came to his mind:

> I remembered having read, ten years or so earlier, Hans Selye's classic book, *The Stress of Life*. With great clarity, Selye showed that adrenal exhaustion could be caused by emotional tension, such as frustration or suppressed rage. He detailed the negative effects of the negative emotions on body chemistry.
>
> The inevitable question arose in my mind: what about the positive emotions? If negative emotions produce negative chemical changes in the body, wouldn't the positive emotions produce positive chemical changes? Is it possible that love, hope, faith,

laughter, confidence, and the will to live have therapeutic value? Do chemical changes occur only on the downside?

In consultation with his physician, Cousins formulated a program of action to mobilize these positive emotions. His first objective was to reduce the constant pain that kept him awake. He began by viewing episodes of the old television show *Candid Camera*, as well as old Marx Brothers films. The results were immediate.

> It worked. I made the joyous discovery that ten minutes of genuine belly laughter had an anesthetic effect and would give me at least two hours of pain-free sleep. When the pain-killing effect of the laughter wore off, we would switch on the motion-picture projector again, and, not infrequently, it would lead to another pain-free sleep interval. Sometimes, the nurse read to me out of a trove of humor books.

Eventually Cousins improved enough to return to work. By 1979, when he published the best-selling *Anatomy of an Illness as Perceived by the Patient*, he reported that he had become pretty much pain-free. Cousins's explanation for his experiences was straightforward: "The will to live is not a theoretical abstraction, but a physiologic reality with therapeutic characteristics.... What we are talking about essentially, I suppose, is the chemistry of the will to live."

Body-Mind Health: The Psychophysiology of Emotions

Since publication of Cousins's book, investigation of the neurochemistry of emotions has emerged as a major scientific venture. Research in the new hybrid fields of psychophysiology, psychoneuroimmunology, and neuroendocrinology has begun to map the physiological and biochemical connections that link our emotions and the operation of the several bodily systems.

In *The Psychobiology of Mind-Body Healing*, Dr. Ernest Lawrence Rossi detailed the scientific basis for "mind modulation" of the autonomic nervous, endocrine, immune, and neuropeptide systems, and their complex interactions as they work to produce "mind-body healing." According to Dr. Rossi, there are three distinct levels of mind-body communication: between mind and brain, between brain and body, and between cell and gene. Interestingly, the connecting links along these communication pathways do not consist solely of nerves.

> The nerves are there, to be sure...but the nervous system is only the "Johnny-come-lately" in the evolution of mind-body communication. Before life invented nerves to specialize in rapid communication between brain and body in large-size organisms, messenger molecules were the original form of communication. Even today the activity of every single nerve in our body and brain is modulated by messenger molecules. This is the new and profoundly deep insight that makes a modern science of mind-body communication possible.

These "messenger molecules" have also been called "molecules of emotion" by Dr. Candace B. Pert, neuroscientist and pharmacologist at Georgetown University. They comprise the neurotransmitters of the autonomic nervous system, the hormones of the endocrine system, the cytokines of the immune system, and the neuropeptides of the neuropeptide system. These work in tandem in various ways, connecting our feelings and moods with the physiology and functioning of our body and bodily systems.

Scientists have identified pathways between what are called "affective disturbances"—state and trait anxiety, depression—and the onset, progression, and severity of physical disorders. Emotions influence interactions among the nervous, endocrine, and immune systems in response to infection, inflammation, and tissue injury. Psychological conditioning, personality, coping styles, and emotional responses to stress modulate our immunity, up or down, with implications for disease. Commenting upon the wealth of new evidence, an article in the *American Psychologist*, journal of the American Psychological Association, noted that "the study of the psychological modulation of immunity has only scratched the surface of the relationships that probably exist."

Emotions, Health, and Disease

This new science of emotions and health is not just a matter of arcane facts that could interest only a laboratory scientist. There are important implications for each of us—things we can do to improve our emotional state and influence our health for the better.

In *Minding the Body, Mending the Mind,* former Harvard scientist Dr. Joan Borysenko outlined practical means to understand the "emotional mind traps" that subvert our well-being. These traps, which Dr. Borysenko called "the dirty tricks department of the mind," include negative personal beliefs, social beliefs ("shoulds"), insistence on being right, rationalizing, disillusionment, and despair. Each has negative consequences for our emotions or—as is the case with the last two—is itself a negative emotion. Dr. Borysenko's book is a treasure trove of wisdom on how to understand our own emotional style and begin to reframe our responses to things that happen. In so doing, we can develop healthier emotions and attitudes that ensure "freeing the inner physician."

The possibility of using our emotions as allies in promoting health and preventing illness is intriguing and exciting. But the consequences of an established link between emotions and health are serious. There is a dark side to this connection. If emotions can heal and keep us well, they can also make us ill.

Dr. James W. Pennebaker, psychologist at Southern Methodist University, identifies inhibition of emotions as a major health threat. In *Opening Up,* Dr. Pennebaker explained that holding inside the terrible emotional consequences of traumatic events—incest, sexual abuse, a serious accident, widowhood—increases one's risk of serious health problems. But there are things we can do to cope better with such emotions so that they are not automatically translated into physiological and functional declines. According to Dr. Pennebaker, freely expressing our emotions through confiding in others can be a powerful catharsis and aid in recovering from illness. This includes praying—a powerful means of confiding.

Love and Health

Other experts have singled out love as foremost among the human emotions capable of promoting and maintaining health and achieving healing. *The Complete Guide to Your Emotions and Your Health*, published by *Prevention* magazine, explained: "It seems something deep inside our cells responds positively when we feel love. Love appears capable of sparking healthy biological reactions in much the same way as good food and good fitness."

This sounds very much like the language used earlier to describe how positive emotions stimulate mind-body communications that are key to beneficial immunologic responses. The experience of love—given and received—apparently is good for our health.

Dr. Leonard Laskow, physician and author, has discussed the importance of feeling and expressing love for attaining "holoenergetic healing." This he describes as a transformational process that can bring harmony and balance down to the deepest recesses of the self. In *Healing with Love*, Dr. Laskow stated:

> Emotions impel us to express our feelings through our actions, though sometimes we repress our actions. In a healthy state, our thoughts and feelings are aligned and integrated to guide our actions....Our emotional health depends on our ability to be in touch with our emotions, feelings, and thoughts. Having an awareness of their origins and of their effects on us and on others enhances our sense of self.

Dr. Laskow also described how emotions can influence health through psychoneuroimmunologic mechanisms, as well as through effects on the human bioenergy system. This hypothetical network of energy centers and circulatory channels is believed to contain and direct the movement of a vital life force capable of maintaining health and preventing and healing illness. The existence of this system is controversial; the question is explored in greater depth in Chapter 8.

Dr. Bernie Siegel, Yale physician and author of the best-selling *Love, Medicine and Miracles*, has affirmed, "Unconditional love is the most powerful stimulant of the immune system. The truth is: love heals." Through his Exceptional Cancer Patients (ECaP) program,

Dr. Siegel has worked with individuals to help them experience love and other emotions, such as forgiveness, that can mobilize the immune system and engender health.

Research on the direct health effects of love and forgiveness is still in its infancy. The John Templeton Foundation recently funded more than two dozen research studies of forgiveness. Many of these are investigations of physical and mental health. I recently completed data collection for a small clinical study of the health effects of love, funded by the Institute of Noetic Sciences. Results are not yet published, but I found that dimensions of love—such as feeling love for or feeling loved by God or a higher power—was associated with greater self-esteem, higher levels of self-efficacy or sense of mastery, less depression, less physical disability, and greater self-rated health. These results have led me in a recent scholarly article to propose the "epidemiology of love" as a new scientific field.

Love, Worship, and Prayer

A principal means of experiencing positive emotions, especially feelings of love and forgiveness, is by religious worship and prayer. Through the experience of public and private rituals, religion may ease dread and anxiety, reduce tension and aggression, allay fear, and moderate loneliness, alienation, and feelings of inferiority. Many of these negative affects, or feelings, have been found to be risk factors for illness. Religious rituals characteristically use confession, emotional arousal, and other processes to instill feelings of peacefulness, escape, purification, empowerment, or catharsis.

In a review of scientific findings on religious factors in the prevention of hypertension published several years ago, I elaborated on this point: "These positive affects may serve as sorts of psychic beta-blockers or emotional placebos which mitigate the body's attempt to elevate blood pressure. Rituals from pre-modern, Western, and Eastern traditions encompass mental and physical healing rites or procedures which are associated ethnographically with such cardiovascular benefits."

Dr. Michael E. McCullough, psychologist and faculty member at Southern Methodist University, concurs. In a comprehensive review of published research on the health benefits of prayer, he outlined physiological and psychophysiological pathways by which prayer influences health. Dr. McCullough reviewed evidence that prayer may "facilitate improvements in mood tone...leading to a state of peace and calm during prayer and extending into other areas of the life of the pray-er." These emotional benefits, he suggested, may lead to neuroimmunological, cardiovascular, and brain electrical changes—physiological changes that may promote health.

Of course, religion just as easily can, and does, engender less-savory emotions: dread, fear, anxiety, self-loathing. But just as these emotions and states may be risk factors for illness and psychological distress, so the positive emotional effects of religion may be protective against a wide range of negative health outcomes. Such emotional responses to worship, especially feelings of loving and being loved and forgiven, may be powerful sources of health and healing. Through bolstering our resistance to disease and strengthening the body's immunity and ability to maintain a healthy homeostasis or balance, the positive emotions resulting from religious worship can help us to negotiate and overcome the stresses of daily life.

Lessons to Consider

The evidence in this chapter gives rise to our third principle of theosomatic medicine:

PRINCIPLE 3

Participation in worship and prayer benefits health through the physiological effects of positive emotions.

What do these scientific studies linking devotion and prayer to better health tell us about the value of regular worship? What can we learn from research showing that the positive emotions engendered by prayer affect our physiology, even immunity? Are there health consequences of finding ourselves trapped in uncomfortable religious settings or on an unfulfilling spiritual path?

As we have seen, the most personal aspects of our spiritual life have a direct impact on the workings of our body and mind. How we connect to God or the divine, when and where we worship, how and how often we pray—these issues have implications for our happiness and life satisfaction, our ability to physically function, and our capability of coping with life changes, especially as we grow old. Because prayer and devotion create emotional responses within us, our usual patterns of worship go a long way toward shaping our emotional life. Our relationship with God influences how we get along with others, how we respond to stress, how we deal with daily events, and how we feel about ourselves.

Keeping the lines of communication open with whatever or whomever we conceive God to be is among the healthiest things we can do. Naturally, this means different things to different people. We all have our own ways of conceiving of God and relating to God. But no matter how orthodox or unique our style of expressing devotion to the sacred in life, each of us has an innate need for conveying gratitude to the source of all being. Most religious traditions recognize this by providing liturgies replete with structured prayers, poems, and songs of praise. For many people, devotion is best accomplished without words. They express their thankfulness through silent prayer and meditation, allowing feelings of gratitude to wash over them in very personal ways.

Structured or unstructured, public or private, worship marshals emotions that strengthen what epidemiologists call "host resistance." Also known as "constitution," this refers to our innate ability to withstand illnesses to which otherwise we would be susceptible. Finding a style of worship that we are comfortable with can provide us with inner resources that help us to cope with problems, to buffer stress, and to fend off or recover more quickly from illness. Prayer can steel us to better withstand the biological, psychological, and interpersonal threats to our health and well-being. But this ability of worship to engender strong emotional responses can also be our undoing.

Just as positive worship experiences can flood us with feelings of peace, joy, contentment, belonging, and acceptance, undesirable experiences can fill us with fear, dread, and guilt. For some of us, prayer and devotion are not undertaken to express our love of God or out of longing for union with the holy, but for other reasons. These include fear of chastisement by an angry deity, desire to appease a spouse or parent, guilt over real or imagined sins, or a wish to appear socially acceptable. In some theologies, these may be perfectly justifiable reasons to pray and participate in worship. I do not mean to disparage them. But such motivations may be driven more by the hope of fooling God or other people or ourselves than by the desire to unburden a contrite heart. If we give in to negative emotions during this type of prayer, there may be harmful consequences for our health and for our functioning and well-being. We may think we are fooling someone, but we are not fooling our body or mind.

My own perspective is that worship should be an uplifting experience. This is not to say that it is always purely joyous. Sometimes we come to God in thanksgiving for wonderful blessings that have already filled us with contentment. In these instances, it is easy to see how prayer can be emotionally fulfilling, even ecstatic. Sometimes, however, we come to prayer or meditation burdened with a heavy heart or broken spirit. We may be in the depths of despair, lower than we imagined possible. But when we are sincerely motivated and willing to "let go and let God," worship ought to leave us feeling emotionally better off than when we started. One worship service or a single prayer or twenty minutes of quiet reflection may not leave our spirit soaring with the eagles, but God willing, it should not send us sinking any lower. If we find that how we worship is only making us more miserable, then it may be time to find a new way to pray.

Questions to Reflect On

This chapter began with the story of Ruth. Various infirmities and functional problems prevented her from taking part in the worship services she so adored. Sad and depressed over her inability to attend services, she wisely chose to spend her time reading about the importance of a positive outlook for meeting health challenges. Eventually she was able to return to synagogue and once again experience the joy of worshiping with her friends.

Ruth's experiences should resonate with many of us. Older adults, especially, may derive special benefit from regular religious worship, as it may offer a sense of continuity in the face of increasingly difficult life changes, such as functional declines and disengagement from other activities. Public and private devotion and prayer may also provide a source of hope for the future, which could otherwise be uncertain.

Duke University psychiatrist Dr. Harold G. Koenig, in his book *Aging and God*, outlined the benefits of an active religious life for older adults and throughout life. Religion may exert a protective function, epidemiologically speaking, against mental health problems such as depression, anxiety, and attempted suicide. It may also serve as a means of coping with already existing illness, and may hasten recovery from medical problems and from the psychological pain of bereavement.

Maintaining a familiar style of religious devotion is key to preserving one's emotional stability as physical and other changes occur with age. For younger and middle-aged adults, patterns of worship may serve a similar nurturing and conserving function throughout such life changes as marriage, parenthood, moving to a new community, and changing jobs. Prayer and worship may be old friends that trigger in us the same wonderful feelings that have sustained us before in times of need or radical change. Reinforced over many years, these familiar ways of relating to God, the positive emotions they trigger, and their resultant physiological benefits may become as much a part of our life as our physical characteristics and personality.

Reflecting on my own worship experiences, I recognize how going back as an adult to the religious tradition I had drifted from as a teenager reinvited familiar and comforting feelings back into my life. Once I met my wife, I felt especially drawn to return in earnest to a more active spiritual life, both communally and personally. I felt

I had something big to be thankful for, and I also felt, as do many Jews of my generation, a responsibility to help preserve our traditions. Each time I reconnected with one of the various prayers, synagogue rituals, and annual holiday worship activities, I was flooded with emotions—joy, awe, excitement, reverence—that I recalled from childhood. Today, many years after reestablishing a regular pattern of prayer and devotion in my life, I still experience the same emotions, and some new ones. Worshiping God is, for me, an essential part of daily life and a source of inestimable comfort. In trying times, especially, I know that it has helped to keep me balanced and well.

A lot of people surely can relate to what I have described. My experiences are not unique to myself or to newly observant or recommitted adults of any particular faith or spiritual path. Worshiping God or connecting to the divine presence naturally evokes strong feelings in people. These powerful emotions, in turn, can influence us in various ways—mentally and physically—from making us rethink things we thought we knew to heightening particular sensations. The questions that follow can help us explore how our patterns of prayer and devotion can produce feelings that affect our physical and mental well-being.

1. All religious and spiritual paths have their own unique traditions for expressing devotion to God or to the holy. Both across and within particular faiths, individual followers are called to pray and worship in many different ways. How many ways do you find to worship God or your conception of the divine? Through ritual prayer? Through extemporaneous prayer? Through silence and clearing the mind of all words and thoughts? Do you prefer to worship with others or by yourself? Do you have set times for seeking God in this way, or do you talk to God spontaneously throughout the day?

2. What emotions do you experience during prayer? Are they different depending upon whether you have prayed with others, as in a formal service, or by yourself? What kind of feelings do you have when you participate in other types of sacred rituals or activities, such as singing, chanting, lighting candles, or washing the hands? After you have finished praying or meditating, do

you feel differently than before you began? Are you more contented or relaxed? Or are you more restless? Are you happier? Do you have greater peace of mind? How long do these feelings last? Do you look forward to the feelings you get when you pray or meditate?

3. Do you have physical sensations when you pray or engage in worship? Do parts of your body tingle? If you have any ongoing pain, does the pain level diminish? If you practice meditation, have you ever felt awareness of your body fade away, as if you were pure mind or spirit? Do you ever feel God's spirit wash over you or fill you during worship? Do you lose consciousness? Do you experience any unusual feelings, such as ecstasy or perfect joy? When you pray or meditate, do you ever notice any changes in your breathing or your pulse? Afterward, do you feel less bothered by the daily stresses that are usually present in your life? Have you ever noticed any changes in an existing physical condition during or following personal prayer or worship?

4

Religious Beliefs, Healthy Beliefs

Deborah ran the health food co-op in a large town on the East Coast. It was the early 1980s, and everyone she knew was into vegetarianism and what was then called "holistic" health. Deborah had a college degree in biochemistry and a great interest in topics related to nutrition, organic farming, bodywork, and natural hygiene. She also read everything she could about meditation and the lives of Eastern and Western mystics, saints, and spiritual healers. Most of her friends at the co-op had a similar though more superficial interest in such topics, and some of their tastes also ran to unusual phenomena such as channeled teachings, crystal healing, and UFOs. To Deborah's friends, the allure of these things was a part of their fascination with the growing New Age movement. Customers of health food stores, one might think, also would fit this pattern.

This assumption never struck Deborah as accurate. She was naturally friendly and outgoing, and loved to talk to her customers. She would get to know them and learn about their lives and about what brought them, in a metropolitan area with dozens of modern supermarkets, to shop at a small health food co-op. Deborah had discovered that many of her customers were not actually New Agers like her coworkers, but rather were devout members of more orthodox religious traditions. Many customers were especially strict in their devotion and practices, and felt "called" to shop primarily at the co-op.

Deborah got to know customers representing a wide cross-section of traditional faiths. Some were observant Jews whose dedication to an eco-kosher lifestyle included avoidance of dangerous pesticides and purchase of cruelty-free products. Some were Hindus and Sikhs whose diets depended upon fresh fruits and vegetables and foods with wholesome ingredients uncontaminated by animal products.

Some were Seventh-Day Adventists whose belief in the sanctity of the body as God's temple led them to vegetarian and all-natural diets. And others were Quakers or Muslims or evangelical Christians or contemplatives of various stripes, all of whom shared a desire to put only healthy products into their bodies and to help the cause of social justice by supporting the co-op. Many of these same customers also shared an interest in what are now called "complementary" or "alternative" medical therapies, purchasing herbs and castor oil packs and homeopathic remedies for use at home, and receiving care primarily from chiropractors, osteopaths, and naturopaths.

Years later, Deborah received her Ph.D. in public health and became a research scientist. She has continued to study and pursue her interests in both spirituality and natural health. She remains an interested observer in the alternative health care scene, even contributing to an official government report on research in the field. Deborah continues to observe how people's most deeply held beliefs influence their health practices and responses to illness. She has learned that there is no simple formula such as "only New Agers go to chiropractors," "all Jews keep kosher," "no Christians follow a macrobiotic lifestyle," "all Hindus believe in Ayurvedic medicine," or "people who study the Edgar Cayce readings never go to regular doctors." As she observes in her own life, one's spiritual beliefs and life principles indeed influence health and health-related decisions, but they do so in complex ways that are not easily summarized. Deborah hopes someday to contribute to a better understanding of how people's worldviews and resulting health practices affect health and healing.

For some of us, religious rituals such as group worship or private prayer are welcome interludes providing moments of respite in our hectic lives. Although transient, these brief connections to the eternal bring peace, contentment, and health and well-being. Whether enjoyed publicly with others in a religious service, or privately, at home alone or with one's family or friends, regular worship or communication with God may be a source of strength, sustenance, and healing.

For others of us, religious practice is not just a joyful interruption in an otherwise secular life. It reflects a spiritual worldview or belief system that permeates all aspects of our life, influencing what foods we eat, what people we marry, what work we do, and what thoughts we think about ourselves and the world. For such people, their chosen religious or spiritual path is not just a dimension of life, it is a central and defining feature of their entire personality.

Decades of research have shown that personality styles and patterns of behavior, as well as specific beliefs about the world and about health, strongly influence our health-related behavior, use of health care, and actual health. Our personalities and belief systems condition how we define health, respond to health crises, relate to the health care system, and take care of ourselves to prevent illness and promote wellness. This effect of what we believe, who we are psychologically, and how we relate to the world is especially potent for heart disease and depression. Religious beliefs, through effects on health beliefs and psychological characteristics, are potential sources of illness and health.

Doing Religion versus Being Religious

As we have seen, considerable scientific research by myself, my colleagues, and others reveals that religious affiliation, organized participation, and worship undeniably have striking associations with rates of disease and death and with measures of health and well-being. Each of these relationships between a religious dimension and health reflects the benefits of some type of religious behavior. Affiliating with a religion, participating in organized activities, and taking part in worship are behaviors—they are things we do. Each is a way of *doing religion*.

But what about *being religious*? Is there evidence that affirming religious beliefs or living in accordance with particular doctrines, theologies, or worldviews is beneficial for health or overall well-being?

As with religious affiliation, participation, and worship, the answer appears to be yes. Far fewer studies have investigated the potential health effects of religious beliefs compared to the numerous published studies of religious behavior. Most have focused on such dimensions of well-being as life satisfaction and happiness, rather than physical health. Still, the weight of findings shows that endorsing certain religious beliefs is an epidemiologically protective factor, much as is engaging in certain religious practices.

Do Religious Beliefs Promote Well-Being?

In 1994, I was approached by the National Institutes of Health, which offered me a contract to review and summarize existing research findings that linked religious behavior and beliefs to health and well-being in older adults. My final report was prepared as a monograph for the Behavioral and Social Research branch of the National Institute on Aging, later published in a peer-reviewed gerontology journal. Out of seventy-three studies published between 1980 and 1994, eight included at least one measure of religious beliefs whose effects were investigated in relation to physical or mental health. Some of their results were especially striking.

- A retrospective study of 85 older Canadians found that high scores on a Christian Orthodoxy Scale were associated with greater happiness and life satisfaction.
- A nationally representative study found that belief in the afterlife was strongly associated with finding life exciting, a typical question in lengthier scales of well-being. This belief was also strongly related to greater happiness.
- My colleague Dr. Christopher G. Ellison used the same data to examine "existential certainty" (never doubting one's religious beliefs). This was by far the *strongest* determinant of life satisfaction.

What Do You Think about God?

Other studies have taken more creative approaches to investigating effects of religious beliefs. These emphasize the protective effects of what we believe about God and the divine.

Scientists from Penn State University examined the effect of specific beliefs about God among 1,400 middle-aged Pennsylvanians. Five questions assessed belief that there is a God, that "God knows our every thought and movement," that "God controls everything that happens everywhere," that religion is "better than logic for solving life's important problems," and that to "build a good society" people need "divine or supernatural help." A high score signified "belief in God as a controlling, caring force," and strongly predicted overall life satisfaction, in both sexes. High scores were also associated with greater satisfaction with one's community, job, and even marriage.

An extremely interesting study, conducted by a UCLA social scientist using nationally representative data, took things one step further. Rather than being asked to affirm belief in God, people were asked who God *is*. How respondents characterized God had a lot to say about their well-being and health. Results confirmed not just *that* our beliefs about God affect our well-being, but that *how* we believe in God is crucial.

People were asked, "When you think about God, how likely are each of these images to come to your mind?" Twelve choices were given, grouped into three categories: ruler (including master, king, and judge); relation (including lover, mother, father, spouse, and friend); and remedy (including redeemer, creator, liberator, and healer). People most likely to perceive God as a remedy—a being or force that releases them from or resolves problems of living—reported the highest levels of life satisfaction and satisfaction with health. By contrast, those perceiving God as a ruler—through metaphors of hierarchy—reported the least happiness.

Religious Beliefs and the Prevention of Distress

Studies such as these make the case for religious beliefs as potent agents capable of promoting emotional well-being. Certain beliefs—in God or the divine, or in particular religious tenets—can instill feelings of contentment, happiness, and what psychologists call "congruence," a sense that things have turned out as hoped. Other studies have shown that religious beliefs can also help to prevent psychological distress.

A research team from the Vermont Regional Cancer Center and the University of Vermont investigated the religious beliefs of 71 advanced cancer patients. People were asked to agree with statements on belief in God, heaven, hell, the afterlife, a higher power, the meaning of life, the helpfulness of prayer, and related issues.

Strong religious beliefs promoted well-being and provided sympto-
matic relief. Greater belief, across the board, was associated with
greater life satisfaction. Belief in an afterlife and in the helpfulness
of prayer were associated with greater happiness and positive affect,
or outlook, and belief in heaven was associated with less depression.
Belief in a higher power, in an afterlife, and in the helpfulness of
prayer were also associated with less cancer pain.

Studies like these leave little doubt that religious belief is a key
factor in preventing distress and promoting well-being. According
to a team of British scientists who researched the topic closely, religious and spiritual beliefs "may be at least as important as the more
traditional psychological and secular social factors in the illness
process."

Compared to the evidence for religious affiliation, organized
religious participation, and prayer and worship, however, we have
less knowledge about how and in what circumstances religions and
spiritual beliefs affect our well-being, for the following reasons:

1. The studies we have examined point mostly to religious beliefs
   as protective against psychological distress, but not necessarily
   against illness or death due to physical health problems. Not
   that such a preventive effect is not present—we just do not know
   one way or the other. The research has not yet been conducted.
   Epidemiologic studies of religious beliefs, along the lines of
   those described in Chapters 1 and 2, are especially needed. Nevertheless, we do know with considerable certainty that strongly
   held religious beliefs are associated with less distress and with
   greater happiness, positive affect or mood, and life satisfaction.
2. These studies are based primarily on samples of middle-aged or
   older North Americans, most of whom are members of Christian denominations. Some of the beliefs investigated may be
   meaningful only in this context. Again, we really do not know. It
   would be helpful to learn whether a connection between religious beliefs and well-being or health also exists among members of other religions or nationalities, or in younger adults. Dr.
   Neal Krause of the University of Michigan, who conducted an
   interesting study of belief in the Ten Commandments, acknowledges that studies that ask only about belief in familiar Judaeo-

Christian doctrines and laws "obviously do not exhaust all of the basic religious tenets." He suggests that researchers begin exploring the effects of "beliefs that cut across specific faiths," such as that God intervenes to help us through difficult situations, or that God blesses the faithful.

3. Just as we know little about whether religious beliefs influence health or about what beliefs in particular are consistently protective, we are somewhat in the dark on another important issue. We do not yet have a clear understanding of how and why religious beliefs are beneficial in those areas in which we do have solid data, such as for emotional well-being. Nor is there much consensus as to why religious beliefs should be associated with health. As was noted in the previous three chapters, it is one thing to observe a pattern of scientific findings—in this instance, the presence of a positive effect of strong religious beliefs on well-being; it is quite another to offer a reasoned explanation for why such an effect is present.

Links in a Chain:
Religious Beliefs→Healthy Beliefs→Health

Just how religious beliefs affect our health or well-being is a complicated question. I propose that strongly held religious convictions influence our overall well-being by encouraging beliefs about health and illness that themselves are known to be associated with better health or health practices. How exactly this occurs, and in what circumstances, is less certain. As a scientist, I naturally tend to fall back on the tried-and-true excuse that more research is needed. But I will be bold here and present my ideas about what I believe is going on.

It has been suggested that specific religious beliefs shape our ideas about illness and health—that sickness is a punishment for sin, for example, or that health is a blessing from God. These beliefs may have a lot to say about how people who affirm them cope with illness or distress, or even recover, and whether a religious intervention such as prayer is a part of the response. A Duke University study found that "prayer and medical help-seeking are not mutually exclusive," and that relationships among religious and health beliefs and responses to illness are complex. The authors, Drs. Lucille B. Bearon and Harold G. Koenig, concluded that

> religious beliefs are indeed intertwined with older adults' beliefs about their health and physical symptoms. Many older adults see their health and illness as being at least partly attributable to God and, to some extent, open to God's intervention. Such beliefs might impact on a person's health by causing that person to delay reporting symptoms to a health care provider or to be resistant to complying with prescribed treatment regimes, with the expectation that God will do the healing. A more positive consequence could be that a person would find strength and motivation in compliance, reinforced by the sense that God is helping in the healing process. For many people, prayer may complement medical care, rather than compete with it.

Drs. Bearon and Koenig offer a solid take on why there is a relationship between religious beliefs and health or well-being. An additional possibility is just as provocative.

Are Religious Beliefs Similar to Healthy Beliefs and Personality Styles?

In her outstanding textbook *Cultural Diversity in Health and Illness*, Dr. Rachel E. Spector outlined numerous religious beliefs that may affect health-related behavior, use of health care, and even health itself. Some of these were discussed in Chapter 1. Dr. Spector has done much to systematize our knowledge of how particular religious beliefs help mold our beliefs related to health.

In the first edition of her book, in 1979, she detailed specific beliefs related to birth, death, diet, and response to health crises for thirty-two of the world's religious and faith traditions. These included not only the mainstream Protestant denominations (e.g., Baptists, Methodists, Lutherans) but numerous established Christian sects (e.g., Seventh-Day Adventists, Mormons, Christian Scientists), major world religions (e.g., Hindus, Buddhists, Muslims), non-Christian sects (e.g., Bahais, Black Muslims), and various other new religions and miscellaneous traditions (e.g., Spiritualists, Religious Science practitioners, Native Americans). This tour de force, whose centerpiece is a comprehensive ten-page table, is must-reading for all health care professionals.

By the fourth edition of her book, published in 1996, Dr. Spector had expanded her already thorough discussion of the religious beliefs that prescribe and proscribe specific responses to health events. She extended her enumeration of religious beliefs to those addressing abortion, artificial insemination, autopsy, birth control, blood and blood products, euthanasia, healing beliefs, healing practices, medications, organ donations, right-to-die issues, surgical procedures, and visitation. It is impossible to read the material that she has summarized without coming to the conclusion that religious beliefs profoundly shape our perceptions, beliefs, attitudes, and actions related to health and illness, and likely our actual health status as well.

A common theme among health-related religious beliefs, says Dr. Spector, is that religion "dictates social, moral, and dietary practices that are designed to keep a person in balance and healthy. Many people believe that illness and evil are prevented by strict adherence to religious codes, morals, and religious practices."

It is not simply that such beliefs are medical trip wires, violation of which leads inexorably to ill health as a punishment for apostasy or sin. Some religions promote such a view, to be sure, and examples are many. For other faith traditions, though, the prescriptions and proscriptions are canonized in religious belief to provide believers with a road map that will point the way to, if not ensure, the kind of long, productive life thought to result from living in harmony with nature and nature's laws.

In many ways, the distinction drawn between specifically religious and health-related beliefs may be artificial. For the late Protestant theologian Dr. Paul Tillich, spirituality is as much a dimension of health as are the biological and chemical domains. Likewise, while many scientists, myself included, have studied the extent to which religious and spiritual beliefs and practices determine overall well-being, other scholars have asserted that spiritual equilibrium is an essential component of, or may even *define*, well-being.

Religion and Personal Control

For scientists who study health-related beliefs, these intriguing issues are more than just abstract topics for debate in scholarly journals. They have practical implications. In many instances, it may be downright impossible even to distinguish between a religious belief and a health belief.

Consider the different terms that psychologists use to describe people based on what they believe about their health. "Internals" are people who tend to believe that they personally control what happens to their health. "Externals" tend to think that their health results from circumstances beyond their control, such as due to chance or "powerful others." Scores of research studies over the past few decades show that internals are more likely to take care of their health through healthy behavior and appropriate use of health care. Being an external has come to be considered a risk factor for illness.

I first encountered the internal versus external concept while in graduate school. Right away, I was struck by how much this distinction mirrored the contrast between believing in a free will and espousing a deterministic theology, such as Calvinism. The implications for me, a public health student with a religion degree, were provocative and raised many questions. Are internals how they are because they were brought up in a free-will faith, or because they share an innate family characteristic that produces highly confident and empowered people in both the religious and health domains? Are people who attest to beliefs characteristic of externals admitting a lack of control over their health, or are they affirming a theology that might be empowering and health-promoting in other ways? Are there differences in health-related behavior—and religious characteristics—between externals who believe that their fate is controlled by nefarious forces and those whose "powerful other" is a loving God?

Dr. Kenneth A. Wallston, Vanderbilt psychology professor and codeveloper of the internal versus external concept, has shown a strong interest in exploring such issues. His most recent project involves the development and validation of a scale to assess people's beliefs about the role of God in their health. Future medical research using this measure may go a long way toward answering some of the perplexing issues clouding our understanding of how religious beliefs and health beliefs relate to each other and to health.

Religion and Type A Behavior

Closely related to patterns of health-related beliefs are those personality styles or behavioral patterns associated with particular illnesses or health conditions. The most famous is the Type A behavioral pattern, sometimes referred to as the Type A personality. Long believed to represent a risk factor for heart disease (although this view has been tempered in recent years), the Type A or coronary-prone behavioral pattern has been described by Dr. C. David Jenkins, developer of the Jenkins Activity Survey, a measure of Type A, as a "style of living characterized by extremes of competitiveness, striving for achievement, aggressiveness (sometimes stringently repressed), haste, impatience, restlessness, hyperalertness, explosiveness of speech, tenseness of facial musculature and feelings of being under the pressure of time and the challenge of responsibility."

Dr. Jenkins's description of Type A is eerily reminiscent of an earlier description of a certain religious belief system well known to religious scholars. Nearly a century ago, Dr. Max Weber, one of the founders of sociology, first described the "Puritan ethic" of colonial Protestants. In a famous essay published in 1904 and later issued in book form as *The Protestant Ethic and the Spirit of Capitalism*, Weber noted that this "psychological attitude" was common among Calvinists and was characterized by asceticism, competition, a sense of hard work as obligation, frugality, and fierce self-control. This sounds an awful lot like Type A. According to Weber, this Puritan ethic was instrumental in the rise of capitalism. A number of medical researchers note that the similarities between the Puritan ethic and Type A are overt.

Dr. Karen A. Matthews, a renowned psychosocial epidemiologist and investigator into the Type A concept, noted that aspects of this behavioral pattern may reflect "the cultural context of the Protestant ethic." Researchers from the University of Michigan and the University of North Carolina have expanded on this point, noting the strong correspondences between the two concepts.

> Central to the notion of Type A behavior is the Calvinist idea that it is necessary to continue accumulating goods in excess of one's needs. Weber's analysis demonstrates the individual's competitive achievement and sense of time urgency on a cultural level. The belief that work is a manifestation of being "saved" and that salvation is always uncertain promotes the unclear performance expectations, social comparisons with high achievers, and the lack of clear links between efforts and outcomes which are components of the intrapersonal and interpersonal perspectives on Type A behavior.

My former teacher, Dr. Berton H. Kaplan, has elaborated on this theme with a series of questions: "What part does this 'ethic' in fact play in generating Type A personality traits? How does the search for salvation create stress, e.g., harsh discipline of body and senses? How do religious beliefs and practices relate to character structure?"

Recently, an interesting effort was made to test the possibility of a connection between Weber's Protestant ethic and the Type A behavioral pattern. A study of 40 adults by a psychologist at University College London examined associations between scores on the Jenkins Activity Survey (JAS) and measures of beliefs associated with the Puritan ethic. Overall, the Type A score was strongly correlated with the Puritan ethic, as was a subscale of the JAS designed to assess a tendency to be hard-driving.

Religion, Psychology, and Health

Despite the seeming convergence of the Type A pattern with the Puritan ethic, the influence of religious beliefs on rates of illnesses such as heart disease remains mostly unexplored. Although heart disease is the number one killer in North America, Type A behavior is practically a job requirement for tens of millions of North Americans, and the Puritan ethic remains our most homegrown and widespread theological worldview, few scientists have recognized in these connections any meaningful etiology, or cause and effect. Researchers who continue to ignore the links between Type A and Puritanism and among the myriad of religious and health-related beliefs summarized by Dr. Spector are not just overlooking an interesting and theoretically stimulating area of research. They are failing to see what might be a critical factor in the development of illness and a valuable resource for prevention and healing. Our own research spells this out clearly.

Using data from a well-known study of more than 400 air traffic controllers, I explored the relationships among the Type A pattern, religion, and health along with Dr. Jenkins, my graduate school program director, and Dr. Robert M. Rose, who at the time was chairman of the Department of Psychiatry and Behavioral Sciences at the University of Texas Medical Branch. We found that the direction and extent of health effects of Type A characteristics depend upon the religious beliefs of those being studied. We also found evidence of several other interesting connections between religious beliefs and health. Notably, being a Type A individual was a risk factor for physical illness and elevated blood pressure, but only among certain religious subgroups.

The Type A pattern, measured by the JAS, was strongly associated with the occurrence of illness, but only in New England Protestants, a population more likely to possess Calvinistic religious beliefs than our Catholic and nonreligious comparison groups. Among these Protestants, perhaps religious and personality characteristics mutually reinforced each other, to the detriment of health. Among Catholics, who are less likely to possess Calvinistic beliefs, the Type A pattern and illness were not related. Type A behavior was also associated with greater alcohol consumption, but only in Protestants. Among frequently churchgoing Catholics, Type A behavior was actually associated with *less* consumption of alcohol. Once again, being a Type A was a risk factor for a serious health outcome, but only in a group of people ostensibly more likely to endorse the Protestant ethic.

Other results were just as intriguing. One in particular ran counter to decades of research on the Type A pattern and heart disease. We found startling evidence that Type A characteristics are not necessarily an across-the-board risk factor for cardiovascular morbidity. Higher Type A scores were inversely associated with diastolic and systolic blood pressure in atheists and agnostics. That is, Type A behavior was associated with *less* hypertension. Among these folks, apparently, it is the Type B pattern that is the risk factor. We obtained similar results with infrequent churchgoers. Again, among those ostensibly professing few if any formal religious beliefs, the Type A personality style seems to offer protection when it comes to health.

Along with my colleague Dr. Preston L. Schiller, I also conducted a study of the effect of religion on beliefs about personal control. Once again, results confirmed that the theoretical association has a solid basis in fact. Using data from a study of more than 900 Appalachians, we found more "internals" among Mormons and Catholics, adherents of heavily ritualized, behaviorally strict religious traditions. More "externals," by contrast, were found among Presbyterians, a denomination endorsing Calvinistic beliefs and emphasizing the authority of "presbyters," or powerful church elders. People reporting no religious affiliation had the lowest external score—they were least likely to attribute their health to sources other than themselves.

Scientists have also taken note of how religious worldviews promote beliefs about health. Drs. Daniel McIntosh and Bernard Spilka have asserted that the link between them may be primarily "a function of the relationship between religion and control." Affirming religious beliefs that stress the importance of personal responsibility may naturally reinforce internal control beliefs that encourage healthy behavior. By contrast, growing up with religious beliefs that take a deterministic view of life circumstances ("it's all out of our hands") may engender external-type beliefs that discourage preventive health care. The latter ideas, acted on over time by a population, may lead to higher rates or morbidity or mortality; the former, to less illness and better health.

How Our Beliefs and Personalities
Affect Our Health

The idea that our beliefs about health, or aspects of our personality, might influence our health makes sense and is no longer controversial. What we believe about health and how we approach life and interpret our place in the world say a lot about the decisions we make to practice healthy behavior, seek medical care, and take prescribed medications. Our health beliefs and the knowledge that we have about health influence our decision making as well as our commitment to make changes for the better. This much is obvious.

But can our personality determine our susceptibility to particular illnesses, such as heart disease? Do certain personality styles increase or decrease our risk of morbidity and mortality? Are there direct links between healthy belief systems or personalities and epidemiologic rates of disease? The answer to these questions appears to be a guarded yes.

The scientific field that investigates connections between psychological factors and human physiology and pathophysiology is known as psychosomatic medicine. It is about sixty years old, and is distinguished from the much younger field of behavioral medicine, which focuses on the effects of lifestyle and behavior. About twenty years old, clinical behavioral medicine emphasizes techniques that enable people to change their behavior and acquire skills for preventing disease and alleviating symptoms. By contrast, psychosomatic medicine emphasizes the role of beliefs, attitudes, and personality in health and illness. Psychosomatic researchers are more likely to study psychological states and character traits that increase or decrease risk than behaviors like cigarette smoking or alcohol consumption.

The development of psychosomatic medicine grew out of efforts of nineteenth-century psychiatrists, neurologists, and psychologists who believed that illness had its roots, in part, in the psyche. According to a scholarly history of the field, these pioneers sought to "synthesize information from medical and psychiatric practice, psychology, and biology into a coherent theory of the unity of the mind and body that could be applied clinically." Whether such a theory has ever been developed is debatable. There is certainly nothing in the way of a "unified field theory" of body-mind healing.

Still, research on themes central to psychosomatic medicine has blossomed over the past forty years. Entire fields of study have emerged that explore issues related to the hypothesis of a body-mind connection. These fields include health psychology, psychosocial epidemiology, psychophysiology, and some areas of behavioral medicine. Scientific research in these fields has provided support for two key components of the psychosomatic perspective: (1) that "the notions of mind and body refer to inseparable and mutually dependent aspects of man"; and (2) that "certain attributes of functions of the organism, those that [are] called 'psychologic' or 'mental,' constitute a class of causative agents in morbidity." In other words, mind and body interact and influence health and illness.

Dr. C. David Jenkins, a past president of the American Psychosomatic Society, has described psychosomatic medicine as concerned with the interface of "personal characteristics and processes." These he separates into three categories, each of which interacts with the others, and with the natural and sociocultural environments, to influence disease, death, disability, and recovery from illness. One he calls "personal habits and reactive styles," which includes such familiar lifestyle behaviors as smoking, drinking, drug use, diet, and exercise, known to affect our risk of disease (as described in Chapter 1). He also describes two other categories, whose interrelations define the body-mind perspective on health and illness.

The biological dimension of life represents the functioning of the various bodily systems and organs. These include neurologic processes; special senses; endocrine mechanisms; nutrition, metabolism, growth; digestion; respiration; circulation; hematologic-immunologic function; skin and subcutaneous tissue; the musculoskeletal and genitourinary systems; and reproductive function.

The third category, psychological characteristics and processes, is further divided by Dr. Jenkins four ways: (1) perceptions, including awareness and interpretation of events that happen to us; (2) cognitive functions, or mental activities, including accumulated learning, beliefs, and value systems; (3) emotions; and (4) ego functions, such as defense mechanisms, self-concept, and needs.

Does evidence exist that these psychological characteristics and processes, such as our perceptions or beliefs or self-concept, have anything to do with who gets sick or who stays well? For certain conditions and in certain situations, it appears that psychological states and traits can indeed increase our susceptibility to illness or help keep us well.

Type A and Heart Disease

One familiar piece of evidence is the link between Type A characteristics and heart disease. Research in the 1960s and 1970s suggested that the Type A individual, also known as the coronary-prone personality, was at greater risk for cardiovascular illness and death. Epidemiologic research revealed the Type A pattern to be a risk factor for heart attacks, angina pectoris, and atherosclerosis. The Western Collaborative Group Study, conducted by cardiologists Drs. Meyer Friedman and Ray Rosenman, originators of the Type A concept, determined that Type A behavior was an independent risk factor for heart disease, just like cigarette smoking and high cholesterol.

Later research revealed that the Type A concept comprised several dimensions. Two of these, anger and hostility, when analyzed separately, were found to be most responsible for the increased risk of heart disease. Subsequent work led to the original concept of the Type A pattern being called into question, but it sparked considerable interest in anger and hostility. Research on these characteristics of the Type A individual is a mixed bag, only inconsistently pointing to increased risk.

According to Harris Dienstfrey, editor of *Advances: The Journal of Mind-Body Health* published by the Fetzer Institute, these inconclusive results are no surprise. The problem lies in certain assumptions that underlie these concepts.

> The "mind" that the concepts of Type A and hostility both pre-
> sume—and that is presumed by virtually all the concepts that re-
> searchers currently use to link disease to feelings—works on the
> body like this: A person has a certain set of feelings (attitudes,
> goals, emotions, beliefs, self-perceptions) that leads the person to
> react to certain circumstances in the same way, again and again.
> The feelings have an internal physiological effect....
>
> What this view of mind and body leaves out, of course, is the
> "mindful" mind, the mind that regularly gives a particular mean-
> ing to a person's behavior and experience.

In other words, depending upon other personal characteristics, our past history, or the context in which we experience things that are usually health risks, we may or may not suffer the expected conse-quences of a given risk factor. Hostility may in principle be bad for our hearts, and may affect many or most of us in that way. But not necessarily. Consider, for example, the findings of my colleagues and I, described earlier, showing a protective effect of the Type A pattern for hypertension in nonreligious people. Type A, or any other per-sonality factor, may induce disease in some people, and may enhance successful coping in others. Yet, according to Dienstfrey,

> With a concept like Type A—with any concept that presumes that
> an emotion or a behavioral pattern has a single inevitable physio-
> logical effect on the body—such differences do not matter....
>
> But this makes no sense. It is not reasonable that the playful
> competitor, the envious competitor, and the domineering com-
> petitor all experience the same physiological effects from compe-
> tition [one of the central traits of Type A].

It is more reasonable that the health effects of the Type A or any other psychological state come into play only in the presence of certain other moderating influences. According to UCLA psychol-ogist Dr. Shelley E. Taylor, personality factors "exert their impacts on health in interaction with situational variables such as stress." Cognitive factors, such as how people appraise their situation, have a lot to do with whether certain personality styles or characteristics, such as hostility or anger, are pathogenic or adaptive.

An Unusual Experiment

A fascinating experiment conducted over forty years ago demonstrates how one set of cognitive factors—professing religious beliefs—is associated with a psychological state that alters the cardiovascular effects of stress.

Scientists from the University of Pittsburgh and Harvard Medical School subjected a group of 78 healthy male college students to a very unusual experiment. In a laboratory setting, students were exposed to acute stress while measurements were taken with a blood pressure cuff and a ballistocardiograph. These measures, along with pulse, were used to group subjects into two categories: those whose physiological response to stress was similar to what occurs during the infusion of epinephrine, and those whose physiological response mimicked the response to norepinephrine. Epinephrine has vasodilating effects and is a relaxer of bronchial and intestinal muscles. Norepinephrine is a vasoconstrictor and has many opposite effects.

The experimental stressor consisted of subjects being "given arithmetical problems to do in their heads while being hurried and criticized by the experimenter, or they were asked to repeat a story from memory while talking into an auditory feedback device." Subjects were assessed for their "religious conventionalism," measured by a scale of beliefs about the church, the Bible, God, prayer, and similar topics. High scores, according to the researchers, reflected "a conception of God as punishing power figure and of the church as absolute moral authority, as well as a marked emphasis on faith, tradition, and conformity to institutional forms." The results were striking, and very unusual.

Subjects who responded to stress with a norepinephrinelike cardiovascular response had higher religious conventionalism scores than subjects responding with an epinephrinelike pattern (42.94 versus 33.63). The norepinephrinelike responders were also more likely to have parents who were actively involved in church.

Interestingly, these subjects were also more likely to respond to acute stress by directing their anger outward, toward the experimenter. Subjects who exhibited an epinephrinelike response and professed fewer religious beliefs tended to respond by directing their anger inward or through experiencing anxiety.

This unique study suggests that certain religious beliefs may help protect some people from turning their anger in on themselves and creating the sorts of physiological responses known to be associated with stress-related conditions, such as heart disease and ulcers.

The Role of Personality in Enhanced Well-Being

Just as the potential health effects of personality are moderated by cognitive factors such as religious beliefs, personality, in turn, mediates the effects of other risk factors on physical and mental health. One of these is the stress inherent in sudden or severe life changes.

Evidence from a study of nearly 400 Dutch adults shows that the harmful effects of a deteriorating life situation (in terms of housing, neighborhood, finances, interpersonal relationships, job stress, and so on) on ill health and symptoms of distress are worse among people who are highly neurotic, have low self-esteem, or look outside of themselves for the power that controls their life—those whom psychologists call "externals." Among "internals" with low levels of neuroticism and high self-esteem, negative life changes had no effect on health. Personality factors, it seems, can block the harmful effects of stress from exerting its full force on our health.

Additional research has elaborated on how personality factors enhance well-being, increasing levels of wellness in already healthy people. In their outstanding textbook *The Dynamics of Health and Wellness*, psychologists Drs. Judith Green and Robert Shellenberger provide a primer on psychological states and traits that have been found to promote health and prevent illness.

One of these traits is known as "hardiness." As defined by psychologist Dr. Suzanne Kobasa, hardy people are those in whom stress does not lead inexorably to illness. They seem to have common personality characteristics, including an ability to make commitments, a perspective on change as a positive challenge to be welcomed, and a belief that they, rather than an external force, are in control of their lives.

This is similar to the characteristic known as "mastery," or self-efficacy. Sociologist Dr. Leonard Pearlin, creator of the most widely used scale to assess this trait, describes mastery as the degree to which one believes that one's life chances are under one's control. The flip side to mastery is powerlessness.

Another important personal resource with implications for our well-being is self-esteem. In research, this concept is typically defined as "the sum of evaluations across salient attributes of one's self or personality. It is the overall affective evaluation of one's own worth, value, or importance." The most popular way to assess self-esteem is by using brief scales such as the well-known Rosenberg measure, which asks people to agree or disagree with statements about themselves—for example, "On the whole, I am satisfied with myself," "I feel that I have a number of good qualities," and "At times I think I am no good at all."

Religion and Self-Esteem

Studies have shown how these psychological resources may be bolstered by religious involvement, especially among older adults. The research of Dr. Neal Krause, sociologist and public health professor at the University of Michigan, has been instrumental in demonstrating how self-appraisals of worthiness are a function in part of commitment to a spiritual path. According to Dr. Krause's research, it does not seem to matter how levels of religiousness are assessed—by participation in organized church activities, by self-ratings of the importance of religious beliefs, or by how well belief in God helps one cope with problems. Higher levels of each of these are determinants of greater self-esteem.

- Among 500 middle-aged and older adults included in the National Survey of Black Americans, Dr. Krause and Dr.

Thanh Van Tran, a professor at Boston College, found that the greater one's organized religious participation, the higher one's self-esteem.

- Dr. Krause followed this up in a nationally representative sample of more than 400 older African Americans. The higher one's score on a scale assessing importance of "religious or spiritual beliefs in your day-to-day life" and seeking of "spiritual comfort and support," the higher one's self-esteem.

- A nationally representative Louis Harris survey of more than 1,000 older adults asked people whether they agreed that they received "personal strength and support from God" during difficult times, that prayer helps them "cope with the difficulties and stress" of life, and that it is "important to seek God's guidance" in decision making. Dr. Krause found that affirmative answers were associated with higher self-esteem.

Lessons to Consider

The evidence in this chapter gives rise to our fourth principle of theosomatic medicine:

PRINCIPLE 4

Religious beliefs benefit health by their similarity to health-promoting beliefs and personality styles.

What can we learn from findings linking religious beliefs to psychological states or personality traits known to affect health and well-being? Do spiritual worldviews act as a shield, in a sense, against psychological distress in the face of life's stresses and crises? Does affirming religious or spiritual principles provide a source of strength and meaning that can give us confidence to cope with problems?

The research cited in this chapter shows that strong religious beliefs are associated with higher levels of well-being. The reason appears to be the consonance of certain religious beliefs or world-views with personality traits or psychological states known to have favorable effects on mental or physical health. Just like the gasoline we put in our car to make it run, religious beliefs may be the fuel enabling the positive effects of psychological factors to kick in for the benefit of our health. This is an important possibility for epidemiologists to consider. We know that psychological factors affect our health and well-being, but our picture of how this mind-body connection operates is not as clear as for links described in the first three chapters.

In summarizing the evidence favoring the health effects of psychological factors, Dr. Shelley E. Taylor was led to remark, "Research that examines whether or not psychological...factors are involved in health and illness has largely made its point." Perhaps so, but there is much left to learn, especially in relation to the many states and traits and beliefs that have been overlooked in epidemiologic research. We know a lot about such things as Type A patterns, internal or external source of control, and self-esteem, each of which is influenced by religious belief. But we know less, if anything, about how certain other fundamental psychological attributes relate to our health. Are these, too, affected by religion?

Dr. Berton H. Kaplan identifies several overlooked characteristics, including appreciation, honest self-assessment, forgiveness, love, personal courage, autonomy, wisdom, and trust. There is reason to believe, he notes, that each of these "special gifts and talents" protects against the pathophysiological processes that result in symptoms of heart disease. To Dr. Kaplan, these characteristics look a lot like descriptions of Type B traits, the flip side of Type A, and are highly regarded by most great religious traditions.

Religious Beliefs and Psychological Resources

In a recent paper, Dr. Ellison and I described the many ways in which religious beliefs reinforce positive psychological resources that promote well-being and help us cope with stress and illness.

These functions of religious belief operate, at least in principle, as a healthy influence in our lives.

1. Religious beliefs enhance our "sense of intrinsic moral self-worth." Through bolstering feelings of self-esteem and personal efficacy, a function well supported by research findings, as we have seen, religious beliefs can motivate us to practice healthy behavior and engage in preventive health practices.

2. Religious beliefs influence our perception of ourselves in other ways. Through devotions and studies of sacred writings, we "construct personal relationships with a 'divine other' in much the same way that [we] develop relationships with concrete others." Through a relationship with a just and omnipotent divine being to whom we can turn for guidance and solace, we gain a sense of ourselves as valued, cared for, forgiven, and loved unconditionally.

3. Religious beliefs—not just religious practices—"seem to be especially valuable in dealing with serious health problems (both acute and chronic) and bereavement." These are crises for which there may be no immediate explanation that comforts us, and which "challenge fundamental premises of existence (or indeed threaten existence itself)" and undermine our sense of a just world. Strong religious beliefs may fill this void, helping us to reinterpret problems as events that serve a greater purpose or are part of a greater plan. This reappraisal of challenging, frightening, or hopeless situations can help to stabilize troubled emotions and prevent further distress.

4. Religious beliefs shared with like-minded others, such as members of a congregation, study group, *chavurah*, or meditation group, "reinforce basic role identities, role expectations...and role commitments." In simpler terms, a shared spiritual perspective can lend a sense of belonging, purpose, and mission—perceptions vital in dispelling loneliness, providing meaning, and offering a larger context for life activities. Research by the late Dr. L. Eugene Thomas of the University of Connecticut has shown that these perceptions, supported by religious beliefs, are crucial for preventing depression and emotional distress, dispelling the fear of death, and maintaining well-being. According

to published studies, this apparently universal function of religious belief is as true for retired Englishmen as for Hindu renunciates living in India.

Questions to Reflect On

This chapter began with the story of Deborah. With the inquisitive mind of a scholar, she keenly recognized that spiritual and health-related beliefs are often difficult to differentiate. In many people and in many cultures, they go hand in hand. It may even be impossible to label a particular belief as one or the other. Dietary choices, for example, may be motivated by a desire simultaneously to obey God, to respect one's body, and to advance the cause of social justice. These separate motivations may indeed be indivisible.

Deborah's experiences in observing people from across the spiritual spectrum speak to the complexity of how religious beliefs influence health and health practices. It is not a simple matter of certain beliefs leading inexorably to certain types of behavior, such as following a particular diet or frequenting a particular type of doctor. Even behavior as stereotyped as shopping at a health food store, as Deborah observed, or visiting an alternative practitioner or a metaphysical bookstore, for example, does not necessarily imply New Age beliefs. The link between religious beliefs and health-related behavior is not so direct.

Rather, as we have seen, growing up with a particular set of religious beliefs, or adopting them through formal conversion, or simply developing them over the course of one's life can shape our thought processes, our responses to stressful events, our overall sense of ourselves, and even aspects of our personality. It is these psychological adaptations, in turn, that have implications for our mental and physical health.

In my own experience, by affirming my Jewish beliefs over the years, I have become inclined to adopt or change opinions about a number of health-related issues. My beliefs about end-of-life matters especially, such as artificial life support, do-not-resuscitate orders, and cremation, have evolved as I have grown in my knowledge and appreciation of *halacha*, or Jewish law. By influencing behavioral choices that I make every day, my beliefs have affected me more directly as well. I avoid particular foods and food combinations, try to enjoy a day of rest on the weekend, take time for prayer and meditation, and seek to learn as much as possible about how to prevent illness. Each of these activities probably influences my health—definitely my state of well-being—and each in turn is influenced by religious teachings that I do my best to take to heart.

As we have seen, nearly all religions and spiritual philosophies postulate teachings about health, healing, disease, and death. They may not make the same recommendations as do the teachings of my tradition, Judaism, but they all offer guideposts for living. This is as true for Seventh-Day Adventists' endorsement of vegetarianism as for Anthroposophical teachings on the etiologic significance of hunger and thirst; as true for the Hindu belief in the importance of *prana*, or breath, in regulating health as for the Christian Science teaching that only God is to be relied upon for healing.

Religions and spiritual paths also may encourage worldviews that reinforce personality traits or psychological states that increase or decrease susceptibility to illness. The connections between a Calvinist theology and both Type A behavior and the view that one's life is controlled by an external force are prime examples. The following questions can help us to reflect on how our own religious beliefs and worldviews influence our health beliefs and practices— and ultimately our health.

1. Consider taking an inventory of the various teachings of your religious or spiritual tradition that have to do with lifestyle choices, healthy attitudes, and medical care. How many of these teachings have you adopted as your own beliefs? Have you tended to follow them? Ignore them? Follow some but not all, or drop some after a while? How have you chosen what teachings to live by? Do you believe that you must endorse certain such beliefs to be a faithful member of your tradition? Do you ever feel guilty if you violate laws relating to diet, sexuality, personal hygiene, or use of medical care?

2. Do you have any strong beliefs or attitudes regarding doctors, why people get sick, or what we can do to stay well? For example, do you believe that doctors are generally to be trusted? To be avoided? That what we do or how we live has nothing to do with why we get sick? Everything to do with it? Somewhere in the middle? Do you believe we can make changes in our lives to improve our health and our longevity? Can you say whether these beliefs have been influenced in part by what your religion teaches or by what other people in your religion tend to believe? Is this even a consideration for you?

3. Have you ever made a drastic change in your attitude or approach to health because of a religious teaching you were made aware of, or a new spiritual teaching you heard about? Did you notice any difference in your health? In your emotional well-being? If you had been ill, did your change of attitude enhance your recovery in any way? How have these experiences affected your self-esteem or sense of control? Have you ever acted on religious or spiritual guidance to make health-related decisions that you now regret? Does acting in accordance with religious teachings or through inner guidance play a role in how you respond to health challenges? Would you recommend this course of action to others?

5

Faith, Hope, and Optimism

Heloise, in her mid-forties, had taught high school French in a small Midwestern town for over twenty years. She had a devoted husband and a son who had just finished college. She was a mover and shaker in her community, serving on several boards. She was a pious Christian, extremely active in the Episcopal church. Her family was healthy and well-to-do, and she was contented. Heloise, her friends all said, led a charmed life. Then, suddenly, things began to crumble.

In less than a year, one tragedy after another befell her family. Heloise was diagnosed with multiple sclerosis. The symptoms became so bad that she had to stop working. Her husband's business went bankrupt, and he committed suicide. Her son overdosed on drugs, and entered a residential rehab program. Heloise's mother, who lived in England, died after a brief battle with cancer.

Heloise's friends rallied around her, but she assured them that she was all right. By all indications, she indeed was in remarkable spirits. While initially burdened by the sad events in her family, she quickly adjusted after each tragedy and did her best to ensure that life returned to normal. No one ever heard her complain or recount her litany of troubles, as so many people do. She continued with her volunteer activities for the church, as much as her disability allowed, and maintained her board service to several community organizations. She also added new activities, like visiting homebound members of her church and praying with them. It was what Christ would do, she said.

Heloise's continued activity and chin-up attitude in the face of overwhelming trials began to concern some of her friends. They thought she might be in denial. Her doctor, too, was worried at first, and referred her to a mental health specialist for a thorough workup. Yet, despite an almost textbook array of risk factors for emotional distress—disabling illness, widowhood and other family tragedies, loss of employment, sudden decline in financial status, and family history of mental illness and institutionalization on her father's side—Heloise had no clinical signs or symptoms of distress. It hardly seemed possible.

Nearly a decade later, things are about the same. Heloise is limited in her physical activity, but not nearly as much as would be expected. She has spent long periods of time in bed, but is currently on her feet, and by her own account, doing well. This is a good thing, she says, as she has a lot to do.

Heloise has a saying that she is fond of repeating: As long as you are faithful to God, God will be faithful to you. She tells anyone who asks that she is grateful to God for her many blessings, and too busy to dwell on her troubles. Heloise is fond of quoting a verse from the prophet Isaiah: "No weapon that is formed against thee shall prosper" (Isaiah 54:17). She remains an inspiration to her friends and somewhat of a mystery to her doctor.

Religion influences health in many ways. As we have seen, affiliation with a religion can affect how we behave in regard to health, organized religious participation provides fellowship and support, regular worship and prayer stimulate positive emotions, and religious beliefs may reinforce certain psychological characteristics or health beliefs. In turn, considerable research has shown that our behavior, social relationships, emotions, personalities, and beliefs are powerful determinants of health. Each of these links between religion and health is well known and well accepted by scientists. The possibility of a religion-health connection is not as controversial as it might at first seem, as it can be understood in terms of concepts and theories widely accepted by scientists and physicians.

Such a connection makes sense because of the influence of faith on action—because faith typically gets translated into religious affiliation, attendance, worship, and belief. A study showing, for example, lower rates of trichinosis among Jews makes sense because, on average, Jewish faith is more likely to lead to avoidance of pork. These are the obvious health effects of faith. But what about faith alone—simple heartfelt trust in God or a higher force, or the profession of religiousness—irrespective of whether it motivates further spiritual involvement? Can this type of religious expression in and of itself influence our health and well-being?

The idea that religious faith may be a powerful force for healing and for maintaining health and preventing illness is not new. In

1910, Sir William Osler, one of the founding fathers of modern scientific medicine, published an essay in the *British Medical Journal* describing "the faith that heals." The theme was revisited in 1975 by the renowned psychiatrist Dr. Jerome D. Frank. Writing in the *Johns Hopkins Medical Journal*, Dr. Frank noted that not only is faith in God salutary, but faith in one's physician or in medical science may also contribute to the success of medical interventions. Indeed it may not be just the physician's treatments themselves that are responsible for positive results. Rather, according to Dr. Frank, medical treatment may be successful principally because it serves to "mobilize the faith that heals in the patients."

Is There a "Faith Factor" in Health?

If faith can heal, can it also protect against illness and promote health and well-being? That is, are there preventive as well as therapeutic consequences of faith? Is faith an epidemiologically significant factor?

According to Dr. Dale A. Matthews, an internist on the faculty of Georgetown University School of Medicine, faith in God indeed seems to be beneficial for physical and mental health. In his recent book, *The Faith Factor*, Dr. Matthews marshals evidence suggesting that expressions of faith are associated not only with the healing of physical and emotional problems and addictions, but with improved quality of life. This makes sense, he notes, because of the positive functions of faith known to be associated with well-being. These include instilling trust in God and providing a source of ultimate hope.

Studies suggest that it is not just formal professions of faith in God that are beneficial for our general well-being. Simply affirming that one is religious or spiritual is a strong and surprisingly consistent determinant of physical and mental health. Many studies address the issue of religious faith by asking people to rate their level of overall religiousness—to provide a subjective assessment of how religious or spiritual they consider themselves. Response options typically include three or four categories such as "not at all," "somewhat," "fairly," and "very," although the exact wording varies.

According to the late Dr. E. Mansell Pattison of the University of California, Irvine, this question provides a unique psychodynamic perspective on a person's spiritual life that is not attainable through other approaches to spiritual assessment. Questions about religious affiliation and church or synagogue attendance, for example, provide information about observable public behavior. Questions about the content of prayers and patterns of religious devotion elicit information about private experiences unique to each individual. What these types of questions have in common is that both involve the assessment of how or how often people *do* religion.

Information about what has come to be known as "subjective religiousness," however, provides a glimpse into how religious people perceive themselves to *be*. Answers to this type of question provide a summary of the myriad intrapsychic determinations that we make about our faith. These determinations are uniquely our own. Researchers recognize that "How religious are you?" is a question that each of us answers in our own way and for our own reasons. Yet no matter how differently each of us goes about answering such a question, nearly all of us can instinctively provide an answer. For this reason, scientists like to use this question as a quick, summary gauge of people's level of overall faith—just as self-ratings of health are considered the easiest and most reliable way to summarize the complex issue of health status.

Subjective Religiousness: A Resource for Mental Health

Using subjective religiousness as a marker for the strength of one's faith, research has produced quite a bit of evidence that demonstrates benefits for psychological well-being. According to several studies I and my colleagues conducted, there is indeed a faith factor in mental health.

Utilizing the National Survey of Black Americans sample, we examined the effects of subjective religiousness, which had been assessed by three questions. One was, "How religious would you say you are," which was scored in the usual fashion; the other two questions asked respondents to rate the importance of religion in a couple of ways. Results: the more religious people felt they were and the greater the importance they attached to religion, the greater their psychological well-being. Moreover, not only was this a strong determinant of well-being—it was a *stronger* determinant than age and even health.

With the recent availability of longitudinal data from the NSBA, we had an opportunity to reexamine these findings. As described earlier, longitudinal data trace the effects of a particular factor over time, enabling epidemiologists to determine cause and effect better than they can through cross-sectional surveys. In this new study, we examined the effects of subjective religiousness on several measures of well-being, and also on a highly regarded measure of psychological distress, the RAND Mental Health Index.

Greater subjective religiousness was once again associated with greater well-being. People who rated themselves as more religious had greater life satisfaction and happiness, as well as fewer symptoms of depression. Greater religiousness, as measured in the first study wave, led to both greater life satisfaction and greater happiness *over a decade later*. These effects, persisting for many years, are similar to the results we saw in Chapter 2 of organized religious participation. This study showed that being or feeling religious—not just practicing religion—has protective effects that last far into the future.

Results of these studies are consistent and persuasive: more faith, more well-being. Findings are limited, though, to African Americans. We have studied members of another ethnic group, Mexican Americans from Texas, with remarkably similar results. In one study, we assessed subjective religiousness with three response options: "not at all," "not very or somewhat," and "very." More religious people had greater life satisfaction, even after controlling for their health.

In another study, among young men, greater religiousness was associated with less disability. Among their grandfathers, results were just the opposite: there was more disability among the more strongly religious. This actually makes sense. Among older folks, internal appraisals of the strength of one's faith increase in compensation for age-related declines in ability—declines that may, on average, curtail regular participation in organized religious activities. This would result in an inverse association with health. In younger folks, who on average have not experienced as many functional limitations, a positive association between religiousness and health reflects the ostensibly preventive or protective function of faith.

Multiethnic Findings from National Studies

Having identified a protective effect of subjective religiousness among African Americans and Mexican Americans, my colleagues and I were curious whether this finding was specific to members of ethnic minority populations. Both groups are relatively homogeneous, in terms of categories of religious affiliation. Over two-thirds of African Americans are either Baptists or Methodists, and over 80 percent of Mexican Americans are Roman Catholics. On average, their socioeconomic status and access to health care are similar. It could be that the health effects of religious faith are in some way a function of these groups' special circumstances. We decided to replicate our analyses in a more heterogeneous, multiethnic study setting.

Using data from three large, nationally representative studies, we investigated the impact of subjective religiousness on both health and well-being. The exact wording and response categories differed across study samples, but the concepts (health and well-being) were equivalent. In each study, people were asked to rate their religiousness. Solid evidence emerged for religious effects on both health and well-being in two of the study samples.

In the Quality of American Life study of more than 1,000 adults, people who rated themselves as more religious had better health, as assessed by physical functioning, subjective health, satisfaction with health, and presence of health problems. In the Americans' Changing Lives study of over 1,500 adults, more religious people had greater life satisfaction.

Dr. Ellison and I are currently conducting another multisample study, using data from several large regional, national, and international health studies. Our goal is to systematically map the effects of subjective religiousness and other religious dimensions on psychological well-being. This work is not yet complete and results have not yet been submitted for peer-review, so what follows must be taken as tentative. Analyses for one of the major samples are final, however, and results are consistent with our earlier findings.

Using data on more than 1,500 adult Americans collected for the multinational World Values Survey, we examined effects of subjective religiousness, assessed by asking people to affirm being "a religious person," "not a religious person," or "a convinced atheist." This very simple question has the advantage of being straightforward and to the point. So were our results. Those who were more religious reported greater life satisfaction, greater happiness, had a more positive outlook, were less depressed, and had a higher level of emotional balance.

Spirituality and the Importance of Faith

We have found less evidence supporting a salutary role of simple faith in preventing physical illness or in promoting better physical health. This could be due to the types of study populations that we have investigated and the samples that we have used. Other scientists who have explored this issue in different settings using different types of religious measures have been more successful in establishing a connection between faith and physical health.

Several studies have used an interesting measure known as the INSPIRIT scale. This instrument was designed specifically to assess spirituality in clinical settings. According to its developers at Harvard Medical School, the INSPIRIT measures the elements of spirituality, including "a cognitive appraisal...which [results] in a personal conviction of God's existence (or of some form of Higher Power as defined by the person)" and "the perception of a highly internalized relationship between God and the person (i.e., God dwells within and a corresponding feeling of closeness to God)." These constitute a good operational definition of faith, and seem to tap the concept more directly than does asking people to rate how religious they consider themselves.

A study using a random sample of more than 400 family practice patients from Georgia investigated the effect of spirituality, assessed by the INSPIRIT, on an index of overall health. High scores on both were strongly related. Further, when INSPIRIT scores were broken into high-, medium-, and low-spirituality groups, the greatest level of physical pain was found in the low-spirituality group and the least pain in the high-spirituality group.

The original study that developed and validated the INSPIRIT also provided evidence of a connection between faith and health. Investigators were interested in learning whether a currently high level of spirituality exerted a protective effect against frequent physical symptoms ten weeks later.

More than 80 patients at Harvard's behavioral medicine clinic were given both the INSPIRIT and the Medical Symptom Checklist, an inventory of twenty-five symptoms associated with stress-related disorders. Spirituality indeed was a strong determinant of fewer subsequent symptoms, even controlling for patients' symptom level at the beginning of the study. Because these were longitudinal data, we can conclude that spirituality exerts a truly protective effect over time.

Blood Pressure and Strength of Faith

Another way to address strength of faith is by asking people to rate the importance of their religious beliefs, their relationship to God, their religion, or their spiritual life in general. This is a common way to assess religiousness in sociological studies, but it is rarely used in health research. Like subjective religiousness, the INSPIRIT, and similar measures, it nicely taps into the "being" rather than "doing" component of religion. Does placing more importance on religion have implications for health?

Researchers from Duke University and the University of North Carolina, directed by Dr. David B. Larson, studied more than 400 men from Evans County, Georgia, who had been asked, "Quite aside from church going, how important in general would you say religion is to you?" Response options were "very," "somewhat," and "not at all." Affirming the importance of religion prevented high blood pressure. Those who said religion was somewhat or not at all important had an average diastolic blood pressure of 87.2 mmHg. Those who said religion was very important had an average reading of 84.0 mmHg.

In this study, Dr. Larson and his colleagues conducted another especially interesting analysis. They were interested in whether the subjective importance of religion "interacted" with attendance at church services. This methodological term refers to something like a synergism. In other words, the investigators wondered, did strong faith increase the already well-known protective effect of church attendance for blood pressure?

Results compellingly showed that it did. Those who did not feel that religion was important *and* infrequently attended church had the highest average diastolic blood pressure (88.2 mmHg). Those who did not feel that religion was important *but* who nonetheless attended church regularly had a somewhat lower diastolic blood pressure (85.0 mmHg). Those who attended church regularly *and* said that religion was important had a still lower reading (83.8 mmHg). These fascinating results raise the tantalizing possibility that whatever the beneficial health effects of organized religious participation, a high level of subjective religious faith makes them even more pronounced.

Faith, Functioning, and Survival

Other researchers have investigated the health effects of faith as assessed by subjective ratings of religiousness. Their studies, too, show that professing faith has implications for health, and they include evidence of a faith factor in relation to "hard" measures of physical health: longevity, survival after surgery, and prevalence of chronic conditions and functional disability.

Scientists at Harvard and Yale investigated the protective effects of religiousness on death rates over a two-year period in an NIH-funded study of nearly 400 older adults living in Connecticut. Subjective religiousness was assessed as usual, combined into a scale with faith as a source of strength and comfort and attendance at religious services. Because the latter question was included, this is not a pure measure of the "being" dimension of religion, as in the other studies discussed in this chapter. However, the inclusion of the first two questions definitely weighted scores on this scale in such a way that valuable information on the health effects of faith can still be inferred.

Among those healthy at the onset of study, religiousness did not make a difference for longevity. Because they were in good health, their death rate was so low to begin with that it was unlikely that any additional factors would lower it even further. Among those ill at onset, a different picture emerged. In sick men who were not religious, the death rate over the course of the study was 42 percent. In sick men who were religious, deaths were fewer by over half—just 19 percent. In women, results were similar: death rates of 20 percent versus 11 percent. Investigators also examined the religious variables separately; each increased the odds of survival. Religious attendance had the smallest effect, leading the researchers to conclude that it is "unlikely that the benefits of religiousness are predominantly due to the social contacts associated with church attendance."

These results were confirmed in a clinical study at Dartmouth using a sample of more than 200 postsurgical cardiac patients. The same measures were used as in the Connecticut study. Deaths in a six-month follow-up period after open-heart surgery were 11 percent in patients who considered themselves "not at all," "slightly," or "fairly" religious. In those who were "deeply" religious, the death rate was *zero*. Not a single religious patient died. As in the Connecticut study, religious attendance offered significant protection as well, reducing mortality from 12 to 5 percent, but not as dramatically as simply being religious. Religious fellowship by itself is a salient protective factor against illness, as we saw in Chapter 2. But when it comes to one's spiritual life, meaning it from the heart is the best protection of all.

A classic study by Dr. Ellen L. Idler, a medical sociologist at Rutgers University, found that the faith factor works in part by buffering the ill effects of stressful or challenging health circumstances. Dr. Idler is one of the pioneering figures in the field of religion and health. In a study of 2,700 adults from New Haven,

Connecticut, she offered persuasive evidence for two interesting and related effects of religion. First, considering one's faith as a source of great comfort helps to lessen the harmful effects of chronic illness on disability. Second, affirming religiousness reduces the harmful effects of disability on mental health.

According to these studies, strong religious faith matters when it comes to physical and mental health. Research by my colleagues and I has pointed to protective effects against psychological distress, and other investigators have underscored the benefits of faith for health. As we have seen, this positive effect is not limited to one particular ethnic group or population. It also does not matter precisely how faith is defined. Whether we consider self-appraisals of overall religiousness, reports of the importance of one's faith or religion, or summaries of how much spirituality one experiences, the results seem to be the same.

Links in a Chain:
Religious Faith→Positive Expectations→Health

What does faith do for a person? Does faith instill a certain mindset? A perspective about one's life or place in the world? Are people with more faith better equipped in some way to meet challenges without succumbing to stress? To resist the disease-enducing effects of certain exposures or risk factors? Are there particular thought patterns or mental processes associated with faith that are beneficial for health and well-being?

I believe all these questions can be answered affirmatively. I propose that faith benefits physical and mental health specifically by promoting hope, optimism, and positive expectations. These cognitions are, by definition, functions of faith. They in turn influence our health and well-being.

Considerable research in the field of health psychology has explored the healthy effects of such concepts as learned optimism, positive illusions, hope, and positive mental attitudes. This work reveals that our thoughts and attitudes, whether factually true or not, exert a powerful impact on our lives. They influence how we perceive ourselves, function in the world, and feel, emotionally and physically.

In epidemiologic terms, they work to prevent morbidity, diminish negative effects of stress, and aid in recovery from illness.

What Is Hope and How Does It Work?

The implications of simple faith for health and illness are intriguing. Whether or not God or the spiritual dimension is objectively real or true, and regardless of one's religious affiliation, attendance, worship, or belief, merely thinking or affirming that one is religious or spiritual, or simply having faith or trust in God, a higher power, or the tenets of a religion, may benefit our health and well-being. The reason is that religious faith can produce hope.

According to Dr. C. R. Synder, clinical psychologist at the University of Kansas and editor of the *Journal of Social and Clinical Psychology*, hope traditionally has been conceived of by psychologists as a positive expectation. Hopeful thought, in particular, has three components. Dr. Synder calls them "goals," "pathways," and "agency."

> Goals are the targets of mental action sequences.... Goals may be short- or long-term, but they need to be of sufficient value to occupy thought. Also, goals must be attainable, yet contain some uncertainty.
>
> To reach such goals, people need to imagine routes to the desired endpoints. Pathway thinking reflects the person's perceived ability to generate plausible routes to goals (with affirming self-talk messages with some variant of "I'll find a way to get this done!").
>
> A motivational component—agency—is needed to propel people along their imagined routes to goals. Agency reflects the belief that one can initiate *and* sustain movement along the imagined pathways to goals.

Dr. Snyder has described in great detail how goals, pathways, and agency interact to lead people to attach value to desired outcomes. When it all comes together—when we are occupied with a goal that we deem important, we believe that we will find a way to reach it, and we believe that we will be successful in accomplishing it—then we can be said to have hope.

The consequences of hope for well-being are significant. Dr. Synder points to studies suggesting that greater hope is associated with less depression, avoidance of behaviors that prolong recovery from illness, less physical pain in response to stress, and greater health-related knowledge. Any resource that can provide hope merits consideration as a potentially protective factor against physical and emotional illness. One such resource is religious faith.

Faith Breeds Hope

Dr. Harold G. Koenig, Duke psychiatrist and researcher, has outlined precisely how faith promotes hope. Especially among older adults and those who are suffering from health challenges or are at risk of becoming ill, religious faith "provides a mechanism by which attitudes can be changed and life circumstances reframed." Moreover, "The degree of hope and emotional strength afforded by religion to some older adults may far exceed that obtainable from other sources."

Going back to our earlier question, just how does faith instill hopefulness and optimism toward the future? What are the functions of faith and how does it manifest in people, ultimately for the benefit of our well-being?

In his chapter in my book *Religion in Aging and Health*, Dr. Koenig described eleven characteristics of faith, reasons that it may be associated with hope and therefore with mental and physical health:

1. Emphasis on interpersonal relations
2. Stress on seeking forgiveness
3. Provision of hope for change
4. Emphasis on forgiving others and oneself
5. Provision of hope for healing
6. Provision of a paradigm for suffering
7. Provision of role models for suffering

8. Emphasis on sense of control and self-determination
9. Promise of life after death
10. Promise of ready accessibility
11. Provision of a supportive community

Dr. Koenig formulated his model of the ways that faith leads to hope in the context of Christianity and Judaism. But as faith enables us to endure suffering, its connection to hope is probably universal.

In *Problems of Suffering in Religions of the World*, religious scholar Dr. John Bowker described how each of the world's major religions accounts for suffering and seeks to understand it and alleviate it in its followers. Judaism, Christianity, Islam, Hinduism, Buddhism, Zoroastrianism, and Jainism—even Marxism and Manichaeism—all have theories of suffering, or ways to provide a context for and draw meaning from hopeless situations. Naturally, what is meant by suffering and how it is understood and remedied differ across these traditions. Likewise, what is meant by a good and faithful member of each tradition differs. Still, precisely because the "realities of suffering are common to us all," every religion seeks to instill hope in those who subscribe to its teachings.

For religious believers or the spiritually committed, hope provides a substantial link between active faith and psychological factors in disease prevention and healing. Being hopeful represents a cognitive state or process that mobilizes beliefs and emotions that, as we saw in Chapters 3 and 4, may reduce the risk of illness as well as hasten recovery. Faith, through its provision of hope and positive expectations, is epidemiologically significant.

Religious Faith and Spontaneous Remission

Whether one's faith is based upon illusions or upon truth matters little here. According to Dr. Jerome D. Frank, "expectant faith can be healing, regardless of whether or not it is objectively justified." So long as being faithful instills hope, then even "miracles" are possible. The thousands of pilgrims to Lourdes and other shrines attest to this fact.

Spontaneous Remission, an annotated bibliography published by the Institute of Noetic Sciences, cites *1,385* medical journal articles reporting cases in which cancer and many other serious chronic diseases seemed to miraculously disappear following treatment believed to be inadequate, or even with no treatment at all. These included remission of cancerous tumors of the lip, oral cavity, and pharynx; digestive organs and peritoneum; respiratory and intrathoracic organs; bone, connective tissue, and soft tissue; female breast; skin; genitourinary organs; eye, brain, nervous system, and endocrine glands; and lymphatic and hematopoietic tissue.

Also documented were remission of infectious and parasitic diseases; endocrine, nutritional and metabolic diseases, and immunity disorders; diseases of the circulatory system, blood, and blood-forming organs; nervous system, sensory organ, and mental disorders; respiratory system diseases; digestive system diseases; genitourinary system and pregnancy and childbirth-related disorders; diseases of the skin, subcutaneous tissue, musculoskeletal system, and connective tissue; and injury-related disorders.

Because current biomedical theories are incapable of making sense of such findings, the compilers of the bibliography, Caryle Hirshberg and the late Brendan O'Regan, offered more than two dozen hypothesized "psychospiritual mechanisms" as explanations for these remissions, one of which they termed "faith/positive outcome expectancy." Although faith and the hope it engenders are subjective states, apparently they are sufficient to cause the eradication of signs and symptoms of disease and the reversal of pathogenic processes.

Some physicians and scientists who are married to a worldview in which such things are impossible may never be willing to accept the existence of a faith factor in health. No matter how many epidemiologic studies are conducted or how many more hundreds of case reports are published in peer-reviewed medical journals, it will never be enough.

For example, on the basis of negative findings from a small, nonrandom sample of cancer patients from a single hospital in Pennsylvania, an editor of the *New England Journal of Medicine* felt compelled to declare, as recently as 1985, that "belief in disease as a direct reflection of mental state is largely folklore." Apparently, the compilers of the spontaneous remission bibliography hallucinated the thousand-plus published cases. It is as if fifty years of research in psychosocial epidemiology, psychosomatic medicine, behavioral medicine, psychoneuroimmunology, psychophysiology, health psychology, medical sociology, medical anthropology, and social psychiatry never existed.

Other doctors and researchers, more open to embracing new ideas, recognize that being a good scientist or healer means being willing to consider new allies in the cause of healing and to welcome opportunities to explore new factors that may prevent illness and promote well-being. This is how science and medicine ultimately advance. Good physicians and scientists know this implicitly. Dr. Viktor Frankl, Holocaust survivor and one of psychiatry's greatest figures, said it best in his classic *Man's Search for Meaning*: "When a patient stands on the firm ground of religious belief, there can be no objection to making use of the therapeutic effect of his religious convictions and thereby drawing upon his spiritual resources."

Placebos: Transmuting Hope into Health

A commonly heard maxim is that we create our own reality. According to this widely shared view, our beliefs about ourselves and the world can indirectly—and perhaps directly—affect our lives and health for better or worse. In extreme form, this simple maxim often becomes, "Our thoughts are 100 percent of the cause of all disease." While few people likely agree with this, most of us probably affirm that our beliefs about situations to some extent shape our reactions and responses. Dr. Norman Vincent Peale's famous "power of positive thinking" has strongly influenced generations of Americans. Optimism, hope, good expectations, and positive mental attitude are characteristics of a healthy frame of mind, and no doubt benefit our overall well-being. But is it possible that the ways in which we perceive the world have more concrete effects?

In her book *Positive Illusions*, Dr. Shelley E. Taylor asked a provocative question: "Does optimism promote health?" Dr. Taylor, professor of psychology at UCLA, proposed that optimism benefits health in two ways. "Functional optimists" can assess the future, identify health risks, and take necessary steps to prevent illness, such as engaging in healthy behaviors. Others see themselves as "invulnerable to health risks," and neglect healthy behaviors. This type of self-deception Dr. Taylor called "unrealistic optimism." The relationship between functional optimism and health seems apparent, but remarkably, she noted, unrealistic optimists may also be at a decided health advantage. "Research concerning the relationship of optimism to physical health is in its infancy, and relatively few investigations have been undertaken to this point. However, what evidence exists suggests that optimistic people may be somewhat healthier."

Some might think that the unrealistic optimists would rather hide their heads in the sand than face the possibility of future illness due to some risk factor in their family history. These folks, we are led to believe, do themselves a great disservice by refusing to acknowledge the risk and seek proper preventive care. Dr. Taylor summarized studies that show that this is not necessarily so. Optimistic people, even those at considerable risk, report fewer symptoms, recover more quickly from surgery, and meet with greater success in alcohol treatment programs than pessimists. What she called "creative self-deception" may be protective against illness. How can this be? Dr. Taylor suggested that the best explanation "for the beneficial impact of unrealistic optimism on health is the powerful and widely documented placebo effect."

The placebo effect has been subjected to increasing scientific scrutiny in recent years. It no longer is seen as just a mysterious anomaly, but now is viewed as a normal physiological response whose biochemistry is becoming much better understood. Dr. Taylor explained:

> How does the placebo effect occur? Our stereotype involves some nearly magical process whereby a person thinks she is going to get better after ingesting a placebo, and either does or thinks she has. In fact, the placebo effect is not purely psychological. People do not get better simply because they think they are going to get better.

Rather, believing that one will get better releases a number of chemicals in the body that may actually promote healing.... Some placebos may stimulate the release by the brain of endorphins, naturally produced bodily chemicals that typically reduce pain and improve mood, at least temporarily. If placebos also promote the release of these chemicals, and research evidence suggests that at least some placebos do, then they likewise may produce a feeling of greater physical comfort and emotional well-being.

According to Dr. Andrew Weil, University of Arizona professor and best-selling author, placebos can produce concrete physiological effects that directly affect our health. Whatever orthodox medicine or drug therapy can do, a placebo can do just as well. In *Health and Healing*, Dr. Weil explained:

There is no direct physical response of the human body to any therapeutic procedure that cannot occur with equal form and magnitude in response to an inert placebo. Placebos can relieve severe postoperative pain, induce sleep or mental alertness, bring about dramatic remissions in both symptoms and objective signs of chronic disease, initiate the rejection of warts and other abnormal growths, and so forth.

No surprise, then, that placebos have been called a "hidden asset in healing." How can we access this apparently universal and all-powerful force for health promotion, disease prevention, and healing? According to Dr. Weil, "Any person will respond to a placebo given under conditions that galvanize that individual's belief."

Clearly, a key to both understanding and making good clinical and preventive use of placebos is the identification of beliefs that engender hope and optimism. Perhaps the richest source of hopeful beliefs and positive expectations is found in the holy scriptures of the world's spiritual traditions.

Promises of Hope in the World's Scriptures

The holy writings of the world's religions are replete with messages promising health and protection to the faithful. Both Torah—the

Hebrew Bible—and the Christian New Testament, for example, contain passages promising health benefits to believers. Those who take these messages to heart may have increased resistance to disease, decreased risk of depression and emotional distress, and hastened recovery from illness. This is because faith leads to hope, and hope has physiological consequences.

A brief survey of the Bible reveals messages of hope that cross the stages of the natural history of disease and address a variety of health outcomes. For example, there are passages that promise the primary prevention of disease. This is defined by epidemiologists as measures that promote health, offer specific protection against disease, or establish barriers to disease agents in the environment. Primary prevention protects people who currently are well but are believed to be at some risk. For example: "If you will heed the Lord your God diligently, doing what is upright in His sight, giving ear to His commandments and keeping all His laws, then I will not bring upon you any of the diseases that I brought upon the Egyptians, for I the Lord am your healer" (Exodus 15:26).

Other scriptural passages suggest that faith offers secondary prevention against illness. This is defined by epidemiologists as measures that prevent the spread of disease, prevent disability, or cure or heal disease outright. Secondary prevention addresses the condition of people who already suffer from illness. For example: "You shall serve the Lord your God, and He will bless your bread and your water. And I will remove sickness from your midst" (Exodus 23:25).

The scriptures of other religious traditions also provide examples of this theme. Buddhist, Taoist, Muslim, and Hindu sacred writings all speak to the rewards of faithful living. Faith—in God, in a higher power, in the divine presence, in the tenets of one's tradition—offers comfort, solace, and mitigation of suffering. Through its provision of hope and its encouragement of appropriate behavior, faith is a pathway to emotional equilibrium and general well-being.

> By faith, by virtue and energy, by deep contemplation and vision, by wisdom and by right action, you shall overcome the sorrows of life (Dhammapada 144).

Following the way from the start he may be said to accumulate an abundance of virtue; accumulating an abundance of virtue there is nothing he cannot overcome (Tao Te Ching 59:137).

Allah is all-sufficient for the man who puts his trust in him.... He will bring ease after hardship (Qu'ran 65:3–7).

Those who ever follow my doctrine and who have faith, and have a good will, find through pure work their freedom (Bhagavad Gita 3:31).

For the devout believer, such scriptures represent powerful promises that, taken to heart, may become self-fulfilling prophecies. Whether religious affiliation, participation, worship, or belief are health-promotive or not, as discussed in Chapters 1 through 4, *expectation* of a benefit from religious observance may contribute to greater well-being, psychological or physical.

Such a blessing delivered to the faithful may naturally result from the link between religious observance and wholesome living. Or, as many devout believers affirm, it may be due to divine grace or the supernatural intercession of God. But even if, heaven forbid, there were no such thing as God, mere faith in God's existence may be enough to promote health and prevent or even cure illness. Independent of all the other health-giving factors discussed in this book, hope and expectation seem to be capable of miracles. This is amply supported by both scientific evidence and theory. There *is* a faith factor in health.

Lessons to Consider

The evidence in this chapter gives rise to our fifth principle of theosomatic medicine:

PRINCIPLE 5

Simple faith benefits health by leading to thoughts of hope, optimism, and positive expectation.

What can we learn from findings linking religious faith and subjective religiousness or spirituality to health and well-being? Given the ability of faith to provide hope, and of hope to influence our state of mind and even the functioning of our body, what does this suggest about the public health significance of positive expectations? Is absence of faith a risk factor that threatens the health of people and populations?

One of the difficulties in communicating epidemiologic findings to nonscientists is the challenge of translating observations that emerge "on average" into personal recommendations. Epidemiologically significant factors—whether they increase risk or offer protection—are determined by statistical relationships identified in large-scale studies of populations. As explained in the Introduction, just because studies show clearly that cigarette smoking and alcohol consumption, for example, are risk factors for heart disease, cancer, and other chronic illnesses, doesn't mean everyone who smokes or drinks will become sick, or that those who don't indulge will be immune from sickness.

A maxim of epidemiology is that our state of health or illness at any given time is a function of a combination of all possible risk and protective factors that can come into play. Epidemiologists divide these factors into three categories, and call this model the "epidemiologic triangle." Some factors are related to pathogenic agents (bacteria, viruses, parasites, toxic chemicals), some to the environment (physical, sociocultural, interpersonal conditions), and some to the "host" (personal characteristics). This last category includes medical history, nutritional status, heredity, physiology, behavior, and psychological states and traits—our thoughts, emotions, and personalities. Where we stand in each of these categories, and how these factors interact with each other, ultimately determine our health. Further, the combination of factors that produce a given result in one person may be dramatically different in another.

These are important caveats in understanding what the presence of a faith factor in health means and does not mean. As with the other agent, environment, and host factors more familiar to physicians and medical scientists, findings presented in this chapter do not suggest that faith is sufficient for prevention or healing of all disease. No factor that we know of fits that description. Maintaining good health and well-being, and preventing illness and distress, are the result of the convergence of many factors. Nor is faith likely a necessary factor in health promotion and disease prevention. Tens of millions of people who are neither religious nor spiritual go about life in excellent health.

What the findings presented in this chapter do suggest is simply this: faith deserves a place at the table in discussions of factors known to prevent illness and promote health and well-being. Faith deserves to take its place alongside family history, health-related behavior, stress, environmental exposures, and all the other factors that we recognize as important for health. Faith is not a magic bullet—but neither is any factor. By excluding faith from scientific discussions of the determinants of health, and from discussions of factors that may be clinically significant in some people, we arbitrarily rule out a potentially powerful ally in reducing distress and promoting health.

Dr. Ian Wickramasekera, a past president of the Association for Applied Psychophysiology and Biofeedback, Stanford professor, and one of the pioneers in the field of psychophysiology, minces no words in his endorsement of the importance of faith for scientists and clinicians: "I believe that understanding the mechanisms of faith, the placebo effect, and learning how to systematically use the power of the expectancy and the memory of prior healings is one of the most important long-term goals for health care in the 21st Century."

Questions to Reflect On

I began this chapter by talking about Heloise. After a happy and seemingly charmed existence, her life became a nightmare of tragedies. One of these was a crippling illness. Bolstered only by her faith in God, she refused to curtail her church activities and sink into self-pity. Years later, nothing has changed: she is still physically limited to some extent, but her mood remains radiant and she is undeterred in fulfilling what she sees as her duty to serve others.

Heloise's story is exceptional. But it differs only in degree, not in kind, from the stories that some of us could tell. Not many of us have had as many challenges and in such quick succession. But we all know people who have maintained their health or spirits in the face of physical disabilities or incredibly debilitating life circumstances.

Why some people stay well, or get well, and others do not is mostly a mystery. One person flourishes, the other does not. There may be few differences in their diet, physical activity, or use of alcohol or tobacco. There may also be few differences in their access to good physicians or medications, in their personal or family health histories, in their environmental or occupational exposures, in their supportive and nurturing relationships, in their experience of positive emotions, or in their expression of healthy beliefs and psychological characteristics. How then do we explain differences between them in physical and mental health?

In their book *Remarkable Recovery*, Caryle Hirshberg and Marc Ian Barasch addressed this question specifically in relation to survival with cancer and other serious diseases. They interviewed scores of people, all with fascinating histories. Some told amazing stories of "miraculous" healings and spontaneous remissions. Other stories not as flashy, but nonetheless remarkable, were of people who had continued to live and be well, inexplicably, despite prognoses that seemed to promise otherwise.

In looking for a common thread, Hirshberg and Barasch sought to understand just what explained these people who were anomalously well. They surveyed findings from studies of many of the same factors explored in this book: personality styles, emotional states, health beliefs, social relationships, psychoneuroimmunology, psychophysiology. In the end, what emerged was more than just a single answer. This is what one would expect in light of our knowledge of the epidemiologic triangle. There are many possible reasons for why people get well or stay well, and the combination of reasons differs among us.

Through interviews with their subjects, however, the authors found that certain themes kept emerging, supported by scientific research findings. One of these themes was the presence of a hopeful and optimistic attitude. Hirshberg and Barasch discussed the results of research which found that 90 percent of a sample of oncologists had seen evidence in their practice that hope and optimism "were of significant benefit to treatment."

This jibes with my own experiences and probably those of most scientists and physicians who have explored this topic. Often I have been with health professionals and the talk has turned to inexplicably well people. I have never spoken with a physician or nurse who did not have a firsthand account of a patient whose faith, hopeful thoughts, or optimistic attitude seemed to play a beneficial role in his or her state of physical or mental health. Many doctors have stories to tell about themselves, but because the topic is considered off-limits in some quarters, their own tales of remarkable recovery or perseverance are untold. This is a great shame, and is quite unnecessary.

As this chapter has documented, the beneficial influence of faith and hope is both well demonstrated and what epidemiologists term "coherent"—consistent with current knowledge about psychological factors in etiology, the natural history of disease, and prevention of illness. The stories of each of us—about the salutary role of faith, hope, and optimism—contribute to the growing database of evidence supporting a faith factor in health. The following questions can help us to reflect on how faith in God or a higher power affects our state of mind and our attitudes toward the future, and ultimately our well-being.

1. Consider the ways in which you experience and express religious faith or a personal sense of spirituality. Do you consider yourself religious? Do you consider yourself not necessarily religious, but spiritual? How do you distinguish between the two? Are you both? Would you say that you have a strong faith in God or a higher power? What does it mean to you to have faith? Does it mean that you trust in God? That you expect God always to be there for you? That you believe in or affirm the teachings of your religion or spiritual tradition? Is faith, for you, about something else entirely?

2. Because of your faith, do you believe that you are more hopeful, in general? More optimistic about the future? Do you believe in

God or a holy or divine presence that knows you and cares about you? Do you expect that God or the universe hears your prayers and responds in some way to your needs? Does your faith give your life a sense of purpose? What do you think your life would be like if you did not have any faith?

3. Do you feel that your faith in God or your commitment to a spiritual way of life makes you a stronger person? Have you ever experienced a time of illness when, you believe, a positive attitude helped to hasten your recovery? Have you ever known someone whose faith instilled a degree of hope that saw them through a physical or emotional challenge in a way that their physician could not explain? What about the opposite—has negative thinking ever helped to make you or a loved one sick? What did you, or they, learn from the experience? In your experience, are faith and optimism an integral part of the "whole armor of God" (Ephesians 6:11) that can shield someone, at least in part, from the harmful effects of stressful circumstances?

PART 3

God, Spirit, and the Future of Medicine

Parts 1 and 2 have presented evidence that public religious participation and private spiritual expression benefit our health. Through behavioral, social, and psychological functions, religion and spirituality alleviate distress and promote well-being, both physically and emotionally. These functions—"active ingredients," as I have termed them—are well accepted by medical science. There is growing evidence, however, that religion also influences our health through other pathways, the discovery of which is at the cutting edge of science and still controversial. Part 3 explores the impact on health and healing of mystical and transpersonal means of connection with God.

The first two chapters in Part 3 provide evidence, respectively, for the last two principles of theosomatic medicine:

PRINCIPLE 6

Mystical experiences benefit health by activating a healing bioenergy or life force or altered state of consciousness.

PRINCIPLE 7

Absent prayer for others is capable of healing by paranormal means or by divine intervention.

The final chapter of *God, Faith, and Health* explores the implications of the evidence supporting the seven theosomatic principles. Scientists and physicians are increasingly acknowledging the health benefits of dimensions of our spiritual life—a signal that a new theosomatic model of health, healing, and medicine is emerging.

6

Energy, Consciousness, and Mysticism

Carl was in his eighties, but he looked and felt twenty years younger. A transplanted Texan living up north, he had just retired as a full-time pharmacist, but after his first three days at home he had gone so stir-crazy that he was back at the hospital, volunteering. Carl and his wife had been members of their synagogue for over sixty years. While he had to admit that he enjoyed the social life of his temple, its services did not move him. His spiritual nourishment came from elsewhere.

Back in the early 1970s, when youngsters less than a third of Carl's age were tuning in, turning on, and dropping out, Carl's adventuresome spirit had led him in a most unusual direction. At the suggestion of his daughter, Carl attended a class in transcendental meditation. He took to it immediately, and began a daily meditation practice. Twice a day, for twenty minutes at a time, Carl would sit on the sofa and enter the peaceful void spoken of by mystics. Afterward, refreshed and renewed, he would go about his business with ten times the energy of other folks his age.

One day, Carl began feeling a sharp pain on his right side across from his stomach. His doctor diagnosed the problem as gallstones. Neither medication nor surgery were viable options for Carl, and his doctor recommended a treatment that was experimental at the time: using sound waves to pulverize the stones. Carl would have to travel to a special clinic in the next state, but since it meant avoiding surgery, that was just fine with him.

Once Carl was there, doctors determined that he was an ideal patient for this therapy. In fact, they decided to use him as a case subject in an international conference to be held at the clinic. Specialists from all over the world were coming to see the new technology demonstrated, and Carl would be one of the star patients. They sent him home and scheduled his return for two weeks later.

While at home waiting to return for his treatment, Carl continued his twice-daily meditation practice, just as he had done for over a decade. His daughter had told him how meditation could be used to improve health, and Carl thought he would give it a try. He quietly repeated his mantra, entered a blissful state of consciousness, and began to visualize a clear white light coming in through the top of his head, radiating throughout his body, and burning like a laser through the accumulated stones in his gallbladder. Morning and evening for two weeks he kept this up, until it was time to return to the clinic.

Before the assembled medical dignitaries from throughout the world, Carl was wheeled into a room for tests to provide images of the size and location of his gallstones. After the tests were run, he gazed through the window and saw several doctors and technicians discussing the results with great animation. The tests would have to be rerun. Again the same thing happened—doctors and technicians heatedly conferring, this time with looks of confusion on their faces.

*The specialist in charge approached Carl and asked him, with great consternation, "What have you done?" Carl did not understand why the doctor was so upset, and was not entirely sure what he was being asked. So he related the story of his daily TM sessions, the visualizations, the white light, and the blissful consciousness. The specialist was incensed. In front of the visiting doctors, he screamed at Carl, "You ****** up our conference!" Carl, it seems, had completely dissolved all of his gallstones.*

Back in his room, just before being discharged, Carl was visited by a specialist from India, one of the guests at the conference. The doctor smiled and shook Carl's hand. "Don't you worry about what that other doctor said," he reassured Carl. "I'm from India and I know exactly what you did. That was very good."

Today Carl is nearly a hundred years old. A widower, he lives in a large apartment in a first-class retirement facility. He still manages to find the time to sit quietly, eyes closed, bringing in the white light. According to his doctor and everyone who knows him, he is in remarkable health.

We have seen how religious affiliation, attendance, worship, beliefs, and faith contribute to preventing illness and promoting health and well-being. Each defines or reflects participation in the outer paths of spiritual traditions—what scholars call "exoteric" religion. The exoteric features include organized denominations, religious services, officially sanctioned prayers and beliefs, and accepted ways to channel one's faith, and research has shown that they involve behaviors, social relationships, emotions, beliefs, and thoughts that are strongly health-related.

Many people, however, do not consider exoteric religion a viable option for their lives. While they are not outwardly religious, they still would affirm an inner spirituality. This may be nurtured through contemplative or mystical activities—what scholars call "esoteric" religion. They may or may not maintain membership in a congregation, go to services, pray official prayers, hold to beliefs learned as children, or consider themselves formally religious. Yet they may experience the divine or sacred through meditation, personal growth activities, creative arts, bodywork, or just being with loved ones or in nature.

For many adults whose religious coming-of-age coincided with the social upheaval of the 1960s, the human potential movement of the 1970s, and the growth of Eastern and New Age beliefs in the 1980s, esoteric spirituality rather than exoteric religion best defines their spiritual life. Daily meditation or incorporation of contemplative elements into traditional rituals, more so than weekly church or synagogue attendance, is the most typical expression of this spiritual path. Such activities may result in the experience of transcendent or mystical states, an altered state of consciousness, and a sense of union or connection with God or the divine.

As with more traditional forms of religious behavior, scientists have investigated expressions of inner spirituality. Moreover, studies have documented the health and physiological effects of meditation and other esoteric practices, as well as of mystical states of consciousness. Research into numinous, or spiritually elevated, states resulting from esoteric spiritual practices is an exciting frontier for the epidemiology of religion. While purely epidemiologic research in this area is still lacking, scientific findings from other fields such as psychology, neurology, anthropology, and sociology are beginning to answer important questions about mystical experience and its relationship to our well-being.

Investigating Mystical Experience

When an epidemiologist like me first explores a new factor such as mystical experience, proposed to be of some significance for health, several basic questions are asked in sequence:

1. We begin by describing patterns of the factor in the general population. This is called descriptive epidemiology and consists of asking "what," "who," "where," and "when." What is the nature of the factor? Who exhibits it? Where and when is it most commonly experienced?
2. We then explore the relationship of the factor to relevant health indicators. These can include clinical and laboratory indices; rates and ratios measuring illness, death, risk, and survival; and scales assessing things like pain, overall health, disability, physical and psychological symptoms, emotional distress and well-being, and quality of life. This is called analytic epidemiology and consists of asking "how." How is this factor related to health or well-being?
3. If analytic studies identify a protective or risk factor, the next task is to ask "why." Why is this factor associated with health (or illness)? This means searching for factors that I have called "active ingredients."

In the first five chapters, we have explored the how and why of such familiar religious dimensions as affiliation, attendance, worship, belief, and faith. In this chapter, because the realm of the mystical may be less familiar and more controversial, we need to back up and start with a little descriptive epidemiology before addressing the how and why. Several questions come to mind: Are mystical experiences common? What type of people are more likely to have mystical or unusual spiritual experiences? What other factors predict, determine, or correlate with such experiences?

It turns out that experiences variously labeled as "mystical," "paranormal," "spiritual," or "numinous" are surprisingly common. Often these occur alongside or as a result of esoteric religious practices, such as meditation. Other times, they manifest as the fruits of exoteric or more traditional religious worship or spiritual exercises, as in the ecstatic visions and experiences of Roman Catholic, Orthodox Christian, and Hindu saints. But one need not be a saint or mystical adept or initiate to have moments of *samadhi*, or bliss, or to experience an altered state of consciousness.

According to a study of mine, even what are often termed "psi phenomena" occur with considerable frequency in the lives of ordinary adults. Using nationally representative data on 1,481 adults from the General Social Survey, I investigated the lifetime prevalence of unusual experiences that had been inquired about in several rounds of the survey over a period of fifteen years. Over 86 percent of respondents reported having had one or more mystical or paranormal experiences, including déjà vu, extrasensory perception, clairvoyance, contact with discarnate beings, and a feeling of numinous or divine contact such as during an out-of-body journey. Fewer than one of seven adults reported never having had any such experiences. The answer to the question, "Are mystical experiences common?" is an emphatic yes.

I also looked to see whether such experiences have become more or less frequent, and who reports them the most. In comparison with data collected in the 1970s, psi experiences have increased and are more common in successively younger age groups. About two-thirds of adults stated that they had experienced déjà vu and extrasensory perception. Reports of contact with discarnates (e.g., deceased loved ones) increased from 27 percent to nearly 40 percent—almost exactly the same proportion of adults reporting attendance at church every week.

I found that these experiences were reported more frequently by people who were more privately and subjectively religious, but less frequently by people who participate in organized religion, even after controlling for things like age, sex, ethnicity, socioeconomic status, and other dimensions of religiousness. The conclusion was unavoidable: exoteric, institutional religion apparently discourages or depresses the experience of mystical states of consciousness.

Mystical versus Diabolical

Perhaps there are times when this is a good thing. After all, the phrase "mystical experience" covers a lot of ground. Some experiences may be pleasant or even blissful—the *nirvana* of Buddhist and

Jaina mystics; the charismatic Christian gift of being filled with the Holy Spirit, as in the so-called Toronto blessing. Other experiences may be neutral—neither inherently wonderful nor awful, just anomalous. Examples include the brief hypnagogic or hypnopompic states between wakefulness and sleep, or the unusual states of consciousness attained by shamans and healers. But some experiences may be downright unsettling, terrifying, or even dangerous.

A disturbing Canadian study of 120 female students bears this out. Researchers at Carleton University in Canada conducted a fascinating assessment of what they termed "diabolical experiences." They administered a twenty-six-question scale assessing four types of experiences: "1) sensing the presence of an evil spirit; 2) the sense of being acted upon by an evil presence; 3) the sense of being intimately assaulted and terrorized by an evil spirit; and 4) being given messages from Satan, being overtaken by him or being used as his agent." The scale consisted of statements of past experiences (e.g., "On occasion, I have felt as though an evil spirit was tempting me," "I have had an intimate encounter with an evil spirit or Satan which left me with a feeling of terror," "At times I have been tempted by the Devil"), which were rated as definitely not true, probably not true, probably true, or definitely true "of my own experience or experiences." Results were eye-opening.

Most students, fortunately, reported few diabolical experiences. Over half scored in the lowest quintile of the scale, and over two-thirds were in the lowest third. For those with more of a history of such experiences, there were mental health consequences: the greater number of diabolical experiences, the greater the psychological distress; the fewer such experiences, the fewer symptoms of distress.

What about more positive, nondiabolical types of mystical experience—*samadhi*, blissful consciousness, a sense of connectedness with God or being filled with God's spirit, and the like? And more mundane experiences, such as moments of heightened intuition and extrasensory perception? Is there evidence that these sorts of states are associated with greater well-being?

Is Mystical Experience a Factor in Well-Being?

According to research on this topic, the answer is a guarded yes. While these studies are not truly epidemiologic—large-scale, longitudinal investigations of defined populations—findings do suggest that certain types of unusual mystical experiences are associated with feelings of well-being.

Studies conducted by Dr. James E. Kennedy, at the time a researcher at the Institute for Parapsychology in Durham, North Carolina, have contributed greatly to our understanding of how mystical experiences influence well-being. A couple of his investigations in particular identified the salutary effects of a wide range of unusual experiences, which he differentiated into several categories.

One study examined the separate effects of what Dr. Kennedy termed "transcendent," "psychic," and "anomalous" experiences in a random sample of more than 100 Duke University students. Lifetime occurrence of transcendent experience was assessed by asking whether one "ever had a transcendent or spiritual experience (overwhelming feeling of peace and unity with the entire creation, or profound inner sense of Divine presence)." Similarly, a history of psychic experiences was assessed by inquiring whether one "ever had a psychic experience (ESP, precognition, telepathy, or mind over matter) or out-of-body experience." Information was combined into a scale of anomalous experience.

Results were mixed, but provocative. Neither transcendent nor psychic experiences, nor anomalous experience in general, was related to mental health or to positive or depressed affect. However, all were strongly associated with greater "meaning in life"—finding purpose and satisfaction in one's life. As in other research, greater meaning in life was associated with greater health. Meaning in life was considerably higher in those who had transcendent experiences, psychic experiences, and any anomalous experiences. Further, 91 percent of those reporting transcendent experiences found them to be "valuable or very valuable"; only 2 percent said they were "detrimental or very detrimental."

In a subsequent study, Dr. Kennedy examined changes in people's lives and well-being due to transcendent or paranormal experiences. His sample of 120 people was much older (average age forty-two) than in the previous study, and limited to those interested in parapsychology and believed to have had anomalous experiences. His objective was to investigate whether such experiences led to an increase in certain psychological characteristics. Results showed that they did.

As a result of their experiences, most people reported many positive changes in their lives: 63 percent noted an increase in their sense of connection to others, 59 percent experienced a greater sense of purpose or meaning, 55 percent reported greater happiness and well-being, 53 percent stated that they were more motivated to maintain their health, and 51 percent were more optimistic about the future. Likewise, many detrimental attitudes declined: 40 percent reported fewer feelings of isolation or loneliness, 45 percent had less worry and fewer fears about the future, 47 percent were less depressed or anxious, and 54 percent had less fear of death.

The results of these studies, taken together, point to beneficial results of anomalous or mystical experiences. This seems to jibe with personal accounts of many people who have been through life-altering events that defy conventional explanation: near-death experiences, out-of-body journeys, moments of clairvoyance or clairsentience, brief states of feeling united with God or with all living beings. After such experiences, for many people, life is never the same.

"Normal" Mysticism

Dr. Kennedy's findings have made an outstanding contribution to our understanding of anomalous experiences. These studies, however, leave some questions to explore. For one thing, they do not capture all the varieties of mystical experience, instead emphasizing paranormal occurrences. Also, they draw on samples unlikely to be representative of the general population, notably college students and adults interested in psychic phenomena. The people studied are not typical, and the events reported may be far afield from what most people would consider as "normal" mystical experiences, if such a thing exists.

One very interesting study successfully addressed these concerns. Its results were consistent with what Dr. Kennedy found. This study examined how mystical experiences of Christians related to a "Spiritual Oneness With All" scale, which assessed the experience of unity and completeness (e.g., "I am one with the absolute," "The universe is a living presence"), and a "Positive and Fundamental Change" scale, which assessed constructive behavioral changes (e.g., "Others have remarked about a positive change in me," "The experience has resolved personal problems in my life," "The experience has provided me with a security I never had").

Dr. Bernard Spilka, renowned psychologist of religion and professor at the University of Denver, examined the effects of seven dimensions of "religious mystical experience" in nearly 200 Christian seminary students, church members, and clergy. Christian mystical experiences led to feelings of oneness and connection and to beneficial and lasting psychological changes. Both were found among those whose experiences consisted of greater "sacredness/holiness" (the depth of awe, reverence, and blessedness conveyed by the experience), "presence of God" (the extent to which one was aware of God's nearness), and "joy and bliss" (a sense of peace and a deeply felt mood).

Studies like these show that mystical experiences can have a positive impact on our feelings of well-being. It makes little difference whether we speak of unusual paranormal events, as may occur in students of parapsychology, or profound transcendent experiences, as may occur in devout Christians or non-Christians. The key here may be the context of the experience. Whatever one's religious orientation or spiritual path may be, an experience that resonates within the experiencer as making sense, containing great meaning, and offering direction or redirection to one's life can be a powerful source of psychological growth.

This is true because such experiences of mystical or numinous states, if deeply felt and held to be real and meaningful, can change how we feel about ourselves and our place in the world. Things once important may now seem transient or insignificant. Once experienced, union with the divine, a sense of complete bliss, or a feeling of transcending reality can alter our priorities. Such experiences can stop us on a dime and radically change our life.

There is another way that mystical experiences can change us. Through such experiences, we may gain access to unusual states of consciousness or mysterious energies or forces that might affect the functioning of our bodies thus and our health or resistance to illness. While the presence of such extrasensory pathways remains controversial and their underlying mechanisms hypothetical, many outstanding scientists have pondered the health implications of altered states of consciousness.

Links in a Chain:
Mystical Experience→Altered Consciousness→Health

A serious and interesting article in the British journal *Social Science and Medicine* considered the potentially protective effects of phenomena linked to or defined by altered states of consciousness. The author, Dr. Louise Mead Riscalla, argued that voodoo, ESP, telepathy, and dreams are highly deserving candidates for epidemiologic research.

> In the area of epidemiology, the influence of extrasensory factors upon health could help account for the inter-relationships of various factors responsible for the transmission of disease. Man is vulnerable to the influence of extrasensory factors by his inclination to absorb messages with the consequence that he often inadvertently becomes the victim of subliminal influences and extrasensory or paraconscious perceptions.

Using the framework of the epidemiologic triangle discussed in the last chapter, consciousness-altering experiences can be conceived of as a "host" characteristic that influences health, illness, and well-being. In combination with other host and environmental factors, a person's history of mystical states of consciousness may be a factor to take into account when considering the complex "web of causation" by which all of the myriad influences on his or her health come together.

Yet before profound spiritual experience can take its place in this web—alongside more accepted host factors such as health history, heredity, personality, behavior, and socioeconomic status; and environmental factors such as family relationships, toxic exposures, job satisfaction, and the like—we must show that it deserves to be there. We must identify how such experience affects the human body.

In trying to understand why mystical experiences are associated with well-being, we do not have the luxury of a body of universally accepted scientific data to draw upon. If the active ingredient in the link between mystical experiences and health and well-being indeed has something to do with altered states of consciousness, we are dealing with an area shrouded in much controversy. The existence and phenomenology of such states, and their associated energies or forces believed to be unleashed or accessed, are accepted by some scientists, rejected by others, held to be delusions by some clinicians, and the source of varying degrees of apprehension among traditionally religious people.

Superempirical versus Supernatural

To bring clarity to this issue, my colleague Dr. Harold Y. Vanderpool and I chose the term "superempirical" to define this hypothetical energy or state of consciousness that we suspect is a link between religion and health. We described it as

> A pantheistic...force [that] is tapped by or inherent in religious practices, beliefs, and rituals. This accessible, although presently unmeasurable and ineffable, healing force or energy is attributed many names across various religious and mystical traditions.... While most religious traditions forbid, discourage, or place restrictions on delving into the mysteries of such power(s), others seek to discover and unleash it through occult experimentation, meditation (either as therapy or self-actualization), the recreational or therapeutic use of hallucinogens, or initiation into the mysteries of some school or group.

This definition covers a lot of ground. It is different from what is meant by "supernatural," which refers to those forces originating or operating outside of the natural universe—which is how some religious traditions conceive of God. "Superempirical" refers to those phenomena that occur within the laws of nature but are not empirically provable—yet. Although such concepts as psi phenomena, mystical states, and parapsychology challenge the currently accepted boundaries of physical reality, according to scientific consensus, they may one day be understandable in terms of some yet undiscovered laws of physics.

Referring to such things as superempirical in no way should be construed as an explicit endorsement of their reality. I have written: "This term implies no judgment as to the existence or nonexistence of such energies—just that such energies, if verified to be consistent with their descriptions in numerous writings, are ultimately naturalistic in origin and operation, even if such a 'nature' is somewhat too subtle for most current instrumentation."

Nor should avoiding the term "supernatural" be taken as a license to dabble. Many religious traditions are guarded or discouraging when it comes to the superempirical domain, and perhaps for good reason. In Christianity, altered consciousness is considered a gift of the Holy Spirit (I Corinthians 12:4–11); in Judaism, Kabbalistic practices are discouraged for those unmarried and under forty; in Hinduism, the *siddhis*, or yogic gifts, are the fruits of many years of meditation and not to be actively sought. Metaphysical initiatory orders typically place barriers before those who want to experience such states for their own sake. Temptations and dangers are said to await those who seek such experiences without sufficient preparation, reverence, or grounding, or who wish to use them for worldly gain.

Still, for those who have such powerful experiences, they are decidedly real. Whether intentionally sought through specific practices or experienced as a sacred gift after weeks, months, or years of spiritual questing, mystical states of consciousness connect us to something beyond words. Whatever this something is or is not, there are important implications for the functioning of our bodies. Scientific studies of a variety of spiritual practices have identified physiological correlates of shifts in consciousness. This research establishes the first piece of the link between mystical experience and health and well-being.

Spiritual States and the Relaxation Response

In 1975, in his best-selling book *The Relaxation Response*, Harvard physician Dr. Herbert Benson described physiological changes resulting from techniques used by many people to prevent themselves from becoming overstressed. These techniques bring on "bodily changes that decrease heart rate, lower metabolism, decrease the rate of breathing, and bring the body back into what is probably a healthier balance." According to Dr. Benson, these methods of self-regulation have "always existed in the context of religious teachings." They include Eastern practices such as meditation, Zen, and yoga. The relaxation response is also known in the West in the form of contemplative prayers of Christian monastics, and meditative practices of Jewish Kabbalists and Sufi mystics.

Dr. Benson compared a variety of religious and secular practices on the basis of their capacity to elicit physiological changes associated with relaxation. Transcendental meditation (TM), Zen, and yoga, for example, can lead to reduced oxygen consumption, and decreased respiratory rate, heart rate, and blood pressure, although scientists continue to debate the evidence. Autogenic training and progressive relaxation, two types of medical therapy, lead to some of the same changes and to decreased muscle tension. Other techniques, such as hypnosis with deep relaxation and sentic cycles, produce mixed results.

A common feature of techniques that produce the relaxation response, Dr. Benson found, is an increase in alpha waves. These slower moving brain waves, depicted in electroencephalograph (EEG) readings, "increase in intensity and frequency during the practice of meditation but are not commonly found in sleep." They are linked to rapid learning, stress reduction, lessened pain and symptoms, increased memory, enhanced creativity, personal growth and mind expansion, and, interestingly, mystical experiences. The altered state of consciousness brought about by these techniques is key, according to Dr. Benson, to discovering the how and why of the relaxation response.

Channeling, Prayer, and Brain Waves

Besides meditation and yoga, other spiritual practices have been found to produce altered states of consciousness that can lead to physiological changes. These include unusual activities—trance channeling, for instance—as well as practices more familiar to most people, like private prayer. Neurophysiological results of such experiences have been well documented through research.

A team of anthropologists from Los Angeles conducted a fascinating study of EEG patterns in a group of trance channelers. This activity is "performed in an altered state of consciousness: while an individual is in a trance, an 'other' entity 'channels' through the practitioner's body. Trance channeling could be categorized as a type of 'possession'...[although] trance channels prefer the term 'blending' to describe their trance state as this term connotes harmony and mutual cooperation between the channel and the entity rather than domination of the channel by the entity." Prior EEG studies had been conducted of TM, Zen, and yoga practitioners, but not channelers. Previous anthropological research on trance states had not examined neurophysiology. This study extended scientific knowledge in both directions.

Investigators studied ten trance channelers, five male and five female. They hypothesized that brain wave patterns would change during channeling, but because of a lack of prior research, they were unable to specify precisely how. Results showed that subjects registered significantly more beta, alpha, and theta brain waves during trance than before trance. They also put out more beta and alpha waves during trance than after. It was concluded that there are "definite neurophysiological correlates to the trance state, and furthermore there is some evidence that these correlates may be patterned." Moreover, this pattern is entirely distinct from what emerges in other practices. For example, TM, yoga, and Zen states show increases in alpha; Zen and TM often show periods of increased theta; and large increases in beta are uncommon in Zen and yoga. During trance there were large increases in all three types of brain waves. Channeling, it is clear, can produce a radically altered state of consciousness.

Trance channeling is an unusual activity, to say the least. The profound shift in consciousness required to enable possession by another entity—real or imagined—is hard to describe if one has not experienced the phenomenon. Perhaps it is not surprising that this state is mirrored by marked shifts in neurophysiology. But what about a more commonly experienced spiritual state—entering into prayer? Do brain wave data suggest that praying to God elicits an altered state of consciousness?

A provocative study by scientists at the University of Louisville School of Medicine examined EEG patterns among male and female adults engaging in prayer. Subjects were evangelical Christians, members of the Church of God, a Protestant denomination based in Indiana. They were asked to pray silently in their usual fashion, concentrating on the adoration and praise of God. EEG readings were taken while at rest before praying, during prayer, and again at rest post-prayer. Investigators had hypothesized that electrocortical rhythms would slow during prayer, as research had shown them to do in practitioners of yoga and TM. But they found just the opposite. According to investigators, "There is no evidence of EEG slowing during prayer. On the contrary, prayer appears to be accompanied by a shift in the direction of shorter duration half-waves, or faster EEGs." The pray-ers had actually shifted away from the alpha range and more toward the beta range of brain wave activity—in the direction of normal waking consciousness and hyperalertness. In other words, the state of consciousness of evangelical Christians at prayer was "altered," to be sure, but in a direction quite the opposite of what had been found for practitioners of meditation.

The investigators were perplexed by these findings, but made an interesting observation. They referred to anecdotal evidence that some very highly experienced meditators—folks thought of as spiritual "masters"—often "show an acceleration in frequency of electrocortical activity, particularly during deep meditation." The shifts in consciousness among evangelicals at prayer appear to mimic those occurring in the most advanced Eastern adepts who have spent years refining their meditative practices.

The implications of this last study are clear. If there are beneficial physiological consequences of spiritually altered states of consciousness, they are not just reserved for mystics and adepts. They are available to prayerful Christians, and by extension, perhaps any sincere spiritual seeker who desires to worship or connect with God.

Intrinsic Religion and Absorption

A recent study that my colleagues and I conducted provides a clue as to what is going on here. We offer evidence for a promising theory of why one's inner spiritual life might be associated with states of consciousness beneficial for health and well-being.

Working with Caryle Hirshberg, scientist and author, and Dr. Ian Wickramasekera, Stanford professor and a preeminent researcher in the field of clinical behavioral medicine, I investigated the association between "intrinsic" and "extrinsic" religiousness and the psychological concept known as "absorption." As assessed by the Tellegen Absorption Scale, absorption is a stable personality trait described as openness to experiencing cognitive alterations— "self-altering experiences," as they have been called. This means that people with high absorption are more likely to attain altered states of consciousness. In prior studies, absorption has been associated with mystical and paranormal experiences, hypnotic ability, and changes in physiological markers such as heart rate, blood pressure, and skin temperature.

The concepts of intrinsic and extrinsic (I/E) religiousness describe our motivations for practicing religion or engaging in spiritual pursuits. They derive, respectively, from psychologist Dr. Gordon Allport's concepts of "interiorized" and "institutionalized" religiousness. Intrinsically religious, or spiritual, people show a commitment to their path or faith tradition for sincere reasons having to do with seeking God, truth, and fellowship. They tend to be tolerant and open. Extrinsically religious people take part in religion more for appearance's sake, or for worldly gain or social acceptability. They are prone to prejudice and dogmatism. I/E religiousness has been a major area of research in the psychology of religion for over thirty years. Many validated scales exist, including the Religious Orientation Scale (ROS) developed by Allport.

Our sample comprised 83 adults in a pilot study of recovery from cancer and other life-threatening diseases. Through scores on the ROS, participants were categorized as purely intrinsic, purely extrinsic, proreligious (high on both types of religiousness), or nonreligious (low on both). Our results were stunningly clear-cut. Intrinsically religious people had *over 20 percent higher* absorption than extrinsic, proreligious, or nonreligious subjects, whose scores did not differ. This study identified in intrinsic religiousness one of the few psychosocial correlates of absorption ever found.

Putting everything together, we can hypothesize how intense religious experiences affect our health. Subjectively perceived mystical or spiritual experiences marshal within intrinsically motivated and highly absorptive people the ability to enter altered states of consciousness. Such states elicit neurophysiological changes capable of lessening the harmful impact of stressful circumstances and other risk factors. Deeply meaningful experiences of these types, achieved through sincere spiritual questing or as a perceived gift from God, are a potentially powerful and epidemiologically significant source of protection among certain people. But this is not the whole story. Altered states of consciousness may affect our health in an entirely different way.

Altered States and Subtle Energies

On Easter weekend in 1970, Dr. Elmer Green, a research psychologist at the Menninger Foundation in Topeka, Kansas, began a series of experiments on the unusual self-regulatory capabilities of a yogi named Swami Rama. Dr. Green, widely recognized as the father of biofeedback (a term he coined), directed the program on psychophysiological self-regulation, or voluntary control, at Menninger for many years. Along with his late wife, Alyce, Dr. Green pioneered research into the ability of the mind to modulate or affect physiological parameters such as blood pressure, heart rate, and skin temperature.

After attaching electrical leads to different parts of the swami's body, the Greens turned on their equipment to began monitoring him. In short order, after first explaining what he was about to do, the swami began warming and cooling his hands and dramatically altering the pattern of his electrocardiogram (EKG). The Greens were amazed. That evening at supper, Swami Rama expressed regret that he had not stopped his heart completely, and promised to make amends the next day. After first signing release forms absolving the Greens and Menninger in the event of his death, Swami Rama sat down, closed his eyes for two minutes, and proceeded to enter a state of "atrial flutter" for over sixteen seconds. In this state, the heart oscillates at a rate high enough to shut down its functioning completely. Immediately following this demonstration, the swami stood back up and went about his business.

In a lengthy letter to Dr. Green several weeks later, Swami Rama tried to describe how he had been able to voluntarily self-regulate physiological processes not believed to be subject to human control. The letter was reprinted in the Greens' book *Beyond Biofeedback*. Swami Rama explained:

> It is most amazing that people do not understand the power of mind over body. My effort is sincere and you will see that there is nothing unscientific in it. Of course, I find some difficulty in explaining certain things which I can do, but cannot explain how they are done.
>
> Doctor, meditation alone is real life. There is nothing higher than meditation, that is my experience in life.

In his letter, Swami Rama referred to certain spiritual practices related to meditation, breathing, and visualization and well known to yogis and other adepts of both East and West. These practices are catalogued in the ancient *Yoga Sutras* of Patañjali. Swami Rama also described other demonstrations that the Greens might wish to witness.

After raising the necessary funds, Menninger invited the swami to return, and this time he was observed to alter his brain wave patterns at will. Hooked up to an EEG, he generated increases and decreases in combinations of alpha and theta waves, brain wave frequencies associated with hypnagogic or psychic states of consciousness. Swami Rama could control his brain wave patterns at will, and would first state aloud what he was about to do, like Babe Ruth's famous "called shot" home run in baseball's World Series. As if this were not enough, as an added bonus the swami entertained the Greens by manufacturing subcutaneous cysts and tumors that he made appear and disappear at will.

In Book Three of the *Yoga Sutras*, written over 1,500 years ago, the Indian sage Patañjali outlined a variety of *siddhis*, or supernormal powers, within the capability of anyone with appropriate preparation and discipline. By combining *asanas* (postures), *pranayama* (breathing exercises), *dharana* (intense concentration), *pratyahara* (withdrawal of the gross senses), and *dhayana* (meditation), and using particular visualizations and *mantras* (sounds), the adept is said to be able to effect changes in the form and condition of gross and subtle matter, and in his or her own physiology or health. Formulas are said to also exist for attaining invisibility and superhuman strength, reading minds, even levitating and predicting the moment of one's death. While Western scientists may adopt a "yeah, right" attitude regarding these claims, the ability of yogis to influence their own immediate physiology by altering their state of consciousness is no longer in question.

Science Studies Consciousness, Energy, and Healing

Several years after the Greens' experiments with Swami Rama, a book called *Science Studies Yoga* appeared that cited scores of peer-reviewed scientific papers investigating the ability of yoga and meditation to influence physiological functioning and health. The book was published by the Himalayan Institute, a spiritual retreat center in the United States founded by the swami, and in it mathematician Dr. James Funderburk reviewed research that left little doubt that we can exert conscious control over physiological functions long believed to be involuntary. Dr. Funderburk cited studies showing that we can lower our blood pressure, decrease muscle tension, slow down or speed up our heart rate, and warm or cool our body temperature through yoga or other spiritual practices that alter our state of consciousness or awareness.

In the quarter century since this book was published, the field of applied psychophysiology and biofeedback has become scientifically accepted, and publication of peer-reviewed studies of psychophysiological self-regulation in psychology and medical journals is now common. The Association for Applied Psychophysiology and Biofeedback (AAPB), which grew out of the old Biofeedback Research Society founded by Dr. Green, is a large professional organization whose annual meeting attracts academic scientists and clinicians from around the world.

It has been speculated that one way in which altered states influence physiology and health is by activating a healing bioenergy, or life force. Such a spiritual force or energy has been given many names across cultures and religious, mystical, and alternative medical traditions. These include ether, *prana*, life force, *wakan*, Holy Spirit, *kundalini*, Christ Consciousness, *chi* or *qi* or *ki*, eloptic energy, *baraka*, orgone, *ruakh*, fohatic power, *huna*, odic force, *mana*, second-state energy, *Gestaltung*, the mytogenetic ray, *munia*, the It, *Odyle*, and so on. Over the years, I have found upwards of fifty to sixty names for such a hypothetical force or energy. Not all of these names necessarily denote the same thing. Many Christians might object to equating Holy Spirit with, say, the mysterious orgone energy named by Dr. Wilhelm Reich. Still, most of these terms and their attendant descriptions are probably culture-specific representations of the same spiritual energy.

The idea of a subtle life energy is close to universal. Most of the world's religious and healing systems, now and throughout history, acknowledge such a concept. Only Western biomedicine, it seems, rejects the idea of a spiritual energy or force that heals disease or helps to maintain health and wellness.

In the Ayurvedic medical system of India, this energy, known as *prana*, circulates along channels called *nadis*, located throughout a ghostlike etheric body that encapsulates the physical body but is invisible to the eyes of those in normal waking consciousness. *Prana* is stored in seven major *chakras*, or energy vortices, located in the etheric body along the spine. In traditional Chinese medicine, the life force is known as *qi*, and it flows along meridians, which would be the Chinese counterparts to *nadis*. The meridian system has been mapped out thoroughly for eons, and it resembles the circulatory, nervous, and lymphatic systems with its weblike arteries and branches. A chart of the meridians can be found hanging on the office wall of most acupuncturists and practitioners of traditional Chinese medicine.

As mentioned, most religious traditions restrict access to information about subtle spiritual energy. By contrast, initiation into its mysteries is offered by many orders and brotherhoods. Added to the subtlety or invisibility of such a hypothetical energy, the secretiveness of formal instruction and subjective nature of experiences make scientific verification of health effects of a bioenergy hard to come by, and harder for many scientists to accept. Many scientists, physicians, and clergy working within contemporary scientific frameworks and exoteric worldviews naturally view such phenomena with extreme skepticism.

ISSSEEM and Energy Medicine

This situation is changing quickly. Just as research on psychophysiological correlates of altered states of consciousness has led to their wider acceptance over the past twenty years, so has the study of a potentially healing bioenergy grown into a burgeoning scientific field. Respected scientists debate the interrelationships among subtle energy, consciousness, and other concepts. Others propose sophisticated models of "psychoenergetic systems" or the "human bioenergetic system"—mapping interconnections among subtle energies, physiological systems, *chakras* and meridians, and "extrapersonal" and "transpersonal" states of consciousness. Dr. William Collinge, in his book *Subtle Energy*, has explored the relationship of subtle energies to such spiritual practices as prayer and meditation. The International Society for the Study of Subtle Energies and Energy Medicine (ISSSEEM), located in Golden, Colorado, was founded by Dr. Green and several of his Biofeedback Research Society and AAPB colleagues in 1989 as an interdisciplinary professional organization for study of the basic sciences and medical and therapeutic applications of subtle energies.

ISSSEEM publishes a peer-reviewed scientific journal, *Subtle Energies and Energy Medicine*, with an editorial advisory board stocked with prominent scientists and clinicians; and hosts an annual scientific conference on such themes as "The Future of Energy Medicine: Integrating Science and Spirit," the topic of the 1998 Conference. This organization has worked to advance the study of bioenergy in relation to consciousness, healing, spirituality, and human potential by drawing on research findings and theories from applied psychophysiology and biofeedback, complementary and alternative medicine, parapsychology, physics, and bioelectromagnetic medicine.

The rapid legitimization of biomedical research on altered states of consciousness and subtle energies has been dramatic, but awareness of this work has not yet permeated all fields of science. The presence of AAPB and ISSSEEM has not allayed the fears of many epidemiologists, who apparently are frightened off even by studies examining the health effects of observable and quantifiable religious behaviors such as church attendance or prayer. Studies of the long-term effects of less-measurable phenomena—for example, spiritually induced states of high alpha brain wave activity or improved flow of *prana* after meditation—are not on the agenda of any epidemiologists that I know.

One small reason for optimism: five former AAPB presidents have served as presidents of ISSSEEM, but as 1997–1998 president I was the first head of ISSSEEM who was trained outside of the applied psychophysiology field—namely, in epidemiology. I take it as a personal challenge to convince my colleagues in public health of the importance of investigating the health effects of spiritually induced states of consciousness and their bioenergy-related correlates.

Lessons to Consider

The evidence in this chapter gives rise to our sixth principle of theosomatic medicine:

PRINCIPLE 6

Mystical experiences benefit health by activating a healing bioenergy or life force or altered state of consciousness.

What can we learn from findings that link mystical experiences to well-being? Do the hypothetical mediating roles of altered consciousness and a healing bioenergy or life force offer any clues as to why intense spiritual experiences often precede dramatic changes in health? Are powerful numinous experiences and altered states of consciousness always beneficial? Can they not just as easily be disturbing and promote severe distress?

We have examined evidence in this chapter that mystical or deeply spiritual experiences are associated with reports of greater well-being. As with nearly all the findings presented in this book, this association is based on population-wide data. It is on average, like all epidemiologic or social-science research findings, which means that the relationship we observe between mystical states of consciousness and mental health is an overall tendency. Not everyone who experiences mystical, paranormal, or otherwise anomalous events is equally uplifted; quite the contrary. For some people, intense religious experiences are frightening and unbalancing, and may lead to or reflect underlying emotional or psychological problems.

Sensing a loving presence, such as of an angelic being or a deceased loved one, can be extraordinarily comforting. It is not hard to reason that such an experience, real or imagined, preceded by prayer or meditation or occurring during the dream state, would strongly and positively affect one's well-being. Yet such an experience may also be a hallucination presaging a psychotic episode.

Studies that ask people such questions as "Have you ever felt as though you were really in touch with someone who had died?" unfortunately cannot read people's minds and determine which situation is present. But they can identify groups of people in whom such experiences are more likely to occur.

Context Matters

The noted sociologist of religion Dr. Andrew M. Greeley explored this theme using national survey data. He discovered that reports of these kinds of unusual contacts were significantly more common among widows. Such experiences also were more common among older people and those who perceived God principally as a source of love rather than judgment. Dr. Greeley found in addition that such reports were more frequent among Catholics and Baptists and less frequent among those with no denominational affiliation.

The occurrence of unusual mystical experiences—and spiritualistic encounters are just one example—is apparently a function, in part, of a religious background or spiritual worldview. The same can be said for whether such experiences, even if initially disturbing, are integrating and comforting as opposed to disruptive or signs of psychopathology. This was the conclusion of a study of intense mystical experiences published in the *Journal for the Scientific Study of Religion*. The author, a Finnish theologian, noted that

> a clearly religious belief structure possibly better absorbs and integrates experiences of a negative kind than does a non-religious belief structure. It is possible that a religious individual can more easily handle internal crisis situations and externally-induced immediate situations because he is in possession of an "arsenal" of solution models of a traditional nature for a large number of different real-life situations.

Other studies have come to similar conclusions. Research on the relationship between belief in paranormal experiences and schizophrenic and schizotypic disorders found that it is the *context* of one's beliefs or experiences that makes all the difference.

Belief in such concepts as spiritualism and precognition and psychic powers, which is common in psychotic individuals, may be a positive and adaptive characteristic in sincere believers—for example, members of parapsychological research societies. According to researchers at the University of New England, interpreting unusual personal experiences in terms of equally unconventional beliefs may "represent a cognitive 'defense' against acceptance of the uncertainty of life events, while for others paranormal belief may be indicative of psychopathology."

Other research suggests that the importance for one's psychological stability of having a context for intense spiritual experiences is not limited to believers in the paranormal. A study at Louisiana Tech University found few differences in personality functioning between believers in the paranormal and those believers in the reality of witchcraft and precognition who also held to traditional Christian beliefs (e.g., in God, the devil, heaven and hell, and the afterlife). Having some sort of framework for interpretation, whatever it is, can help us make sense of unusual events without losing our equilibrium.

Because I am an epidemiologist, and neither a psychologist nor a pastoral counselor, I am unqualified to recommend a particular belief system or worldview. Even if I had such credentials, I would not do so. That decision is highly personal and must come from the heart. Science is incapable of providing the information needed to make such a choice. I do believe very strongly, however, that it can be unsettling to chase after unusual spiritual experiences without solid grounding in *some* tradition, religious or secular, that can frame, interpret, and make sense of such things. Radical shifts in consciousness, sudden awareness of a life force (as in *kundalini* awakenings), experiencing gifts of the spirit, and other tastes of the numinous can be powerful signposts along a path of spiritual transformation or self-actualization. And, according to Dr. Joseph B. Tamney, "Self-actualization is a lifestyle"—not just a parlor game. Growth and rebirth are serious matters, with fruits that are not best acquired through trivial pursuit. They may be more meaningful if experienced as moments of grace.

Questions to Reflect On

This chapter began with the remarkable story of Carl. Faced with painful gallstones requiring medical or surgical attention, this octo-genarian relied upon the meditative techniques he had learned years earlier. To the shock—and consternation—of his physician, he visualized a healing energy in the form of white light that seem-ingly obliterated his gallstones. His illness was almost instantly cured and has never come back.

Carl's experience certainly is amazing. Years of diligence at his meditation practice allowed him access to a healing force that changed him physically in a dramatic way. Was this force or energy located within him? Did it come from somewhere "out there"— from God perhaps? Could both possibilities be true? Do such ad-ventures in consciousness depend upon what religion one belongs to or what type of practices one engages in?

Scholars continue to debate whether a common core of experi-ence underlies the many mystical traditions, religions, and cultures throughout the world. Do the experiences of Jewish Kabbalists, contemplative Christian monastics, Sufis, Tibetan Buddhists, and TM practitioners, for example, converge into a set of similar phe-nomena? Or are they entirely divergent and incomparable?

According to philosopher Dr. Mark B. Woodhouse in his out-standing book *Paradigm Wars*, some commentators assert that there is no such thing as a universal type of mystical experience. Every transcendent experience, every altered state of consciousness is unique and has nothing in common with experiences of others in other traditions. On the other hand, many learned figures in psy-chology, philosophy, and religion have identified "a generic core in mystical experiences." Its characteristics include a sense of unity, positive moods, positive changes in attitudes and behavior, feelings of transcending space and time, possessing an inner knowing, and awareness of the paradoxicality, ineffability, and transience of the experience. "No serious student of mysticism would argue that mystical experiences are everywhere the same in every respect," ar-gues Dr. Woodhouse. Still, higher states of consciousness do seem to be experienced and described in similar ways.

As we have seen, mystical or deeply personal spiritual experiences are common features of life for many people. Often inducing altered states of consciousness or awareness of an indwelling life force or energy, these experiences may precede remarkable healings or shifts in health. Through the following questions, we can begin to reflect on our own unique experiences of the mystical, numinous, or divine, and how they have changed our lives.

1. Have you ever had a mystical or seemingly unexplainable experience? Can you describe it in words? Was it preceded by or concurrent with a spiritual practice, such as prayer or meditation, or a religious ritual? Were you alone or with others? Were you afraid while it was happening? Did you think you were dying? Were you excited? Did you feel transported outside of yourself in some way? Have things like this happened to you more than once? Have you experienced life differently since then? Because of your experiences, have your beliefs about the nature of God, the world, or human beings changed in any way? Do you keep a log or journal of your unusual dreams or experiences?

2. During a mystical or anomalous experience have you ever lost consciousness? Did your consciousness shift in some other way—for example, to a state of heightened awareness or sensitivity? To a feeling like being in a lucid dream? To some other state altogether? During such an experience, have you ever felt a subtle energy or life force moving through your body? Did you do anything in particular just prior to having this feeling? Was it enjoyable? Uncomfortable? Did it make you feel more powerful or capable in some way—for example, more knowledgeable or aware or able to heal yourself or others? Has such a feeling of energy flow ever occurred just "out of the blue"—that is, not preceded by any sort of prayer or meditation? Do you believe that such experiences should not be sought but rather left to God to provide or left to occur naturally? What, if anything, do you think these experiences mean?

3. During or after your first mystical or intense spiritual experience, did you feel different in some way, emotionally or physically? Did you notice any changes in your body or in how it

functioned? Have you ever experienced a healing of some type as a result of such an experience? If not a healing, what about a change in your overall level or health or general well-being? Has your health or mood ever suffered as a result of such an experience? Have you ever tried to actively seek out an altered state of consciousness specifically in order to access a healing energy? Were you successful? Do you believe that such health benefits require some sort of special training or preparation to be accessed, or do you think that they are available to all of us? Do you believe that healings of this type come directly from God or that we alone cause them to happen? Do you consider such healings or health-related changes to be a blessing?

7

To Heal Is Divine

A vicious thunderstorm moved over Galveston, dumping blinding rain on the island. Swirling winds made it difficult to walk. Wearing shorts and flip-flops, I raced out the back door of one of the oldest buildings on the campus of the University of Texas Medical Branch. It was a Monday morning, and I was carrying a copy of my doctoral comprehensive exam questions, which were due back typed and completed the following Monday. I was on my way to lunch, then to the library to begin the most arduous and crucial assignment of my academic career.

As I took my first step in the rain, my flip-flops slipped and the wind pulled me down. My back and my arms crashed down on the first cement step, then the second, then the third, and then the pavement. I lost consciousness for a second, and when I came to I had no feeling in my legs. A moment later, soaked to the skin, I was able to move. Several students ran up to me and asked if I was okay. "Yeah, yeah," I mumbled, and barely able to breathe, gathered up my exam papers and made my way back into the building.

When I struggled into the office, the professors and secretaries could see that something was wrong. I collapsed onto a chair and slowly related what had happened. The head of the doctoral program immediately dropped what he was doing and took me over to get X-rayed. Fortunately, my spine was undamaged, but I had cracked a couple of ribs. It hurt every time I breathed, but there was nothing to do except to give me aspirin. The doctor on call told me it would probably take about six weeks for my ribs to fully heal. To add to my misery, I had injured the bursae in both elbows, and my arms were locking up in a half-bent position. That, too, I was told, could take quite a while to return to normal. The director of physical therapy, a fellow graduate student, generously raced over to set me up with special slings for both arms. There was nothing left to do, and I was discharged.

The professor drove me back to my apartment, put me in bed, and made a bunch of ice packs. He said that he would return in a couple of days to check on me. Just as he left, he reminded me that my comps were due in seven days. "I hope this wasn't a ploy to get out of your exam," he joked. I tried to laugh, but it hurt too much. He let me know that if I needed more time it would be arranged, and not to worry about it. He let himself out of the apartment, and I fell asleep.

When I awoke several hours later, I took stock of the situation and realized I was in a pickle. I had an exam to write, but I was trapped in my apartment, too weak to get out of bed, with both arms bent and immobile, and barely able to breathe. Worse, my roommate was out of the country, so how would I eat? I immediately called my folks in Chicago. My mother was a skilled healer, and she belonged to a circle of friends of diverse faiths who met at her house every week for meditation and healing prayer. She also was part of a phone network of people throughout the country who could be mobilized for prayer at a moment's notice.

Within an hour, a couple of dozen people were praying for me, asking God to heal my ribs and arms. Besides my mother and grandfather and a few close family friends, there were transpersonal therapists, Roman Catholic nuns, New Age psychologists, Orthodox Jews, Episcopalian priests, Jungian analysts, yoga teachers, even a few psychics and born-again Christian M.D.s—mostly people I had never met and probably never will. Meanwhile, I closed my eyes and slept through the night.

When I awoke the next morning, without thinking I rolled out of bed and extended my arm to reach for the light, just like any other day. It took a second to realize what I had done, and I fell back in shock. My cracked ribs were almost entirely better. I could breathe fully, I had full upper-body movement, and there was only the slightest twinge of pain when I took my fist and pounded it into my side as a test. My left arm was pain-free and had straightened out, and my right arm (I am right-handed) was functioning at about 90 percent. After midday meditation and a brief nap, I awoke completely healed.

I was now faced with a dilemma. I wanted everyone to know of the apparent miracle that had taken place, an example of the healing power of prayer. However, I was not anxious to run the risk that my hard-nosed, mostly atheist or agnostic professors would assume that I had faked the whole situation to buy a little more time to think about answers for my exam. A six-week convalescence prayed down to a day and a half would have been just too absurd for them to believe. So I settled on a compromise. I would wear one of the slings for about a week, while successfully completing my comps and turning them in on time. Afterwards, I showed up without the sling. I told everyone about the prayer that I had received, and announced that just one week after my fall, I was completely healed.

To a person, my colleagues were surprised that an expected six-week recovery took only a week. Maybe there really was something to this prayer stuff. A one-week healing was remarkable and challenging to accept, but was still within the realm of conceivability. But not a day and a half. I am convinced that if my professors had seen me around town the day following my accident, after they had been gracious enough to offer to extend the deadline for my comps, they would have kicked me out of graduate school.

To this point, I have described the many ways that religion can prevent illness and promote health and well-being. Affiliating with a religion reinforces healthy behaviors, decreasing our risk of disease. Attending services nurtures supportive relationships, buffering effects of stress and heightening our ability to cope. Worshiping and praying produce positive emotions, relaxing us and bolstering the function of our endocrine and immune systems. Adopting certain religious beliefs encourages healthy beliefs and personality styles, motivating wise health decisions. Professing faith stimulates optimism and hopefulness, which are salutary. And ultimately, experiencing a sense of the mystical can lead us into states of awareness that invoke an ability to maintain well-being or attain healing. This would seem to exhaust all of the possible ways by which religion and spirituality can benefit our health and well-being.

But there is one more possibility—namely, that there is a God or divine presence that can choose to bless us in ways that may violate the apparent physical laws of the universe.

Most traditionally religious people in the Western world probably affirm some version of this idea. We may conceive of God in different ways—as fully or partly transcendent, or completely "immanent" (not existing beyond or outside of nature). But most of us who believe in a personal God who created the universe also believe that this loving being or presence can respond to our prayers, even if it is for reasons that we may not completely understand. Surveys show that this belief is common among adult Americans. The idea that the creator of the universe is able and willing to instill wellness, prevent illness, and even heal disease is widely accepted in the West; and variations of this idea are accepted in the East, despite different conceptions of God.

The Healing Power of Prayer

Belief in the healing power of prayer is acknowledged within numerous spiritual traditions. These include established Western religions such as Roman Catholicism, mainline Protestantism, evangelical Christianity, and Judaism. Affirmation of the ability of prayer or focused intention to call forth a divine response for purposes of healing is also found within the writings of many esoteric or metaphysical orders, including Alice Bailey's Lucis Trust, the Theosophical Society, Rudolf Steiner's Anthroposophical Society, Max Freedom Long's Huna Research Associates, and Manly P. Hall's Philosophical Research Society. These traditions differ in their beliefs about what prayer is, how prayer works, when it is and is not answered, and why it can influence our health. But, according to Pierre Marinier, they all acknowledge that prayer, from the perspective of the pray-er, is a "means of access to the cosmic consciousness."

The possibility that prayer for others can promote health or healing can be studied. The conclusion that positive results signify divine or supernatural intercession never can be proven by science. By definition, the concept of the supernatural implies something beyond or outside of the realm of nature. Scientific research requires observation of natural phenomena. Therefore, if there is a God that influences our health in ways that transcend all possible natural forces, no study can ever prove or disprove the fact. The best that we can do in relation to such works of grace is either to accept them on faith or reject their possibility.

This limitation has not prevented researchers from trying to document the healing efficacy of "absent" prayer, whereby pray-er and pray-ee are separated by space and time and do not come into physical contact. The results of their efforts, while empirically unable to prove divine intervention, are nonetheless provocative and challenging.

Can Absent Prayer Heal?

The most famous study of absent prayer, conducted by San Francisco cardiologist Dr. Randolph C. Byrd, was published in 1988 in the *Southern Medical Journal*. In this well-designed randomized, double-blind trial of 393 adult subjects, coronary care unit (CCU) patients who were prayed for by Christian prayer groups outside the hospital did better than patients who did not receive prayer. What made these findings so remarkable was that patients were randomly assigned to the treatment and control groups, neither patients nor hospital staff knew who was in which group, and patients and pray-ers never met. In essence, the study was equivalent to a tightly controlled pharmaceutical trial. This study has received a lot of publicity, and it is merited.

Intercessors were born-again Christians with an active daily devotional life and membership in a local church, either Protestant or Roman Catholic. Experimental subjects were assigned to from three to seven intercessors, who were given only their respective assignees' first name, diagnosis, and general condition. Treatment consisted of daily prayer until hospital discharge. All data were collected in blinded fashion. Results were uncanny. Prayed-for patients, in comparison with controls, had fewer cases of congestive heart failure, cardiopulmonary arrest, and pneumonia, and less need for diuretics, antibiotics, and intubation. These findings, according to Dr. Byrd, "suggest that intercessory prayer to the Judeo-Christian God has a beneficial therapeutic effect in patients admitted to a CCU."

A firestorm of criticism ensued. Subsequent issues of the *Southern Medical Journal* printed letters from physicians with heated comments about the Byrd study. One letter writer criticized the journal and its editor for attempting to return medicine to the "Dark Ages" by publishing this study. Quite the contrary, reasoned a follow-up correspondent, adding, "The *Journal* is to be encouraged in publishing such articles, because objective, scientific assessment of prayer, faith-healers, or what have you is an appropriate endeavor and one in which most readers will be interested."

I agree. Dr. Byrd is to be commended for tackling a controversial and provocative issue with great methodological skill and scientific objectivity. He practically single-handedly brought consideration of intercessory prayer to the forefront of research into body-mind healing and complementary and alternative medicine. This is what good science is all about.

Many other less-known studies of prayer and spiritual intercession have obtained similar results, and not just in humans. According to published reviews, notably the four-volume *Healing Research* by physician Dr. Daniel J. Benor, more than 150 experimental trials exist of the in vivo and in vitro effects of prayer and other spiritual interventions in enzymes, cells, fungi, yeasts, bacteria, seeds, plants, amoebas, and animals. Over half found that the intervention was effective—it healed, promoted health or growth, or prevented sickness or death of the organism.

Prayer and Prayerlike Interventions

Not all of this research is of religious behavior that could strictly be thought of as prayer. According to Dr. Jerry Solfvin, there are studies of interventions termed "mental healing," "psychic healing," "spiritual healing," "nonmedical healing," "shamanic healing," "prayer healing," "miracle healing," "laying on of hands," "paranormal healing," and "magnetic healing." These concepts cover considerable ground and are not necessarily interchangeable. "A wide variety of specific practices and techniques are included, such as passing hands over the patient, invoking the aid of spirit guides or deceased ancestors, praying to God or the saints, administering magical or blessed medicines, or applying some form of mental concentration to 'will' the disease away."

Still, according to Dr. Larry Dossey, most of these studies did investigate effects of prayerlike behavior, even if they used other terms to describe it.

> Part of the problem in identifying work in this field is the lack of agreement on language. Many researchers shy away from using the word "prayer" in favor of a more neutral term such as "distant intentionality." Even though their experiment may actually involve prayer, they often do not use this term in the titles of their papers. If their subjects pray, the researcher may say instead that the subject "concentrated" or applied "mental effort" to produce the effect being studied, or they may use terms such as "mental healing," "psi healing," or "spiritual healing" to describe their work.

In other words, there may be even more published evidence on the healing effects of prayer than current literature reviews have captured.

Taken together, this research covers a lot of territory. Studies have revealed the beneficial effects of prayer and spiritual interventions on physiological parameters such as wound healing, on chronic conditions such as hypertension, on mental illnesses such as major depression, and on infectious diseases such as AIDS. Several studies have been especially noteworthy.

Noncontact Therapeutic Touch

A California researcher conducted a randomized, double-blind, placebo-controlled trial of the effect of Noncontact Therapeutic Touch (NCTT) on experimentally administered subcutaneous skin wounds in 44 male college students. Therapeutic Touch is a modern subtle-energy-based healing technique. It is similar to the ancient practice of laying on of hands, in which the conscious intent of the healer is used to assist the healing process; but with NCTT, *no physical contact takes place.*

Subjects and controls were given a small, full-thickness dermal wound on their deltoid muscle by an M.D. using local anesthetic and a skin biopsy instrument. They were then seated against a wall with an opening that allowed them to pass their arm through to the next room, where an NCTT practitioner practiced her art on subjects but not controls. The experiment lasted sixteen days. Neither the study participants nor the NCTT practitioner nor the M.D. knew the true objective of the research. The M.D. believed that it was a study of Kirlian photography. Treated subjects experienced more rapid wound healing than controls. By day eight, the average wound surface area in subjects was 3.90 mm^2 and in controls it was 19.34 mm^2; by day sixteen, these figures, respectively, were .418 mm^2 and 5.855 mm^2. In fact, by day sixteen, 13 of the 23 treated subjects had a wound surface area of 0.00 mm^2; they were completely healed. None of the controls could say that yet.

Distant Healing and Blood Pressure

Two interesting controlled experimental studies explored the impact of distant healing techniques on blood pressure readings. One study investigated the results of treatment by a group containing Religious Science practitioners; the other examined effects of a group of Dutch paranormal healers.

In the first study, California researchers investigated the ability of eight healers to lower the blood pressure of experimental subjects. Of 96 patients, half were randomly assigned to a control group. Four healers were members of the Church of Religious Science who practiced a four-step prayer called Spiritual Mind Treatment. It consisted of relaxation, "attunement with a Higher Power or Infinite Being," visualization or affirmation that the patient is perfectly healthy, and thanking God or "the Source of all power and energy." The other healers included two Protestant clergy and two other people with strong reputations as healers.

This study was double-blind; neither patients nor physicians knew who were subjects or controls. Healers had only patients' initials, sex, age, health problem, and location. After more than six months, controls had experienced an average drop in systolic blood pressure of about 8 mmHg. Treated subjects, by contrast, had experienced an average decline of 13.8 mmHg.

These results are intriguing, for sure, but of limited clinical relevance. Because systolic blood pressure can fluctuate due to situational anxieties, it is not as good a health indicator as diastolic blood pressure. Can absent prayer affect diastolic and not just systolic blood pressure?

In the second study, a team of medical scientists from University Hospital in Utrecht, the Netherlands, conducted a prospective randomized trial of what it termed "paranormal healing" as treatment for hypertension. A special feature was the random assignment of 115 patients to one of three groups: one receiving laying on of hands, one receiving absent healing, and a control group. The first two groups were treated by twelve members of Dutch paranormal healing organizations. Treatment consisted of a twenty-minute session once a week for fifteen weeks.

Results were inconclusive, compared to the previous study. Still, notable effects were observed. Between the start of the trial and week fifteen, systolic blood pressure declined in all three groups, but more so in the treated groups. Controls declined by an average of 14.2 mmHg, those in the absent healing group by 17.5 mmHg, and those in the laying-on-of-hands group by 19.3 mmHg. Diastolic blood pressure showed a similar trend. Control patients declined an average of 6.7 mmHg, absent healing subjects by 8.6 mmHg, and the laying-on-of-hands group by 9.4 mmHg. Results held regardless of patients taking antihypertensive drugs. One bonus result: patients receiving laying on of hands scored highest on a post-treatment scale of general well-being.

Distant Healing and Mental Illness

Therapeutic effects of absent prayer on psychiatric disorders have also been studied. Noteworthy differences have been observed between treatment subjects and controls.

A researcher at the University of Connecticut Health Center investigated what he termed "distance healing" as an adjunct to standard antidepressant medication in a sample of 40 adult psychiatric inpatients. Patients were randomized into treatment and control groups, and the intervention proceeded in double-blind fashion. Healers and subjects had no contact, and did not know one anothers' names. Patients were assigned to up to four healers.

Healers assigned to patients in the treatment group had been trained in the LeShan meditative distance healing technique. Every day for six weeks, they conducted a session for their respective patients. This involved seeking "to induce through meditation a particular altered state of consciousness for which they had been trained, described as 'nonlocal mind.' While in that state, they included the subject in their minds in a nondirective manner, excluding any other mental content or focus in a state of deep, intense compassion." Following the intervention period, treated subjects had less depression and general psychopathology than controls. Also, the more treatment received, the greater the improvement. The investigator concluded that "the distance healing did exert some therapeutic effect on these patients."

Distant Healing and AIDS

Each of these studies is provocative and provides some, albeit limited, evidence that absent prayer or spiritual intercession has an effect on illness. Because of design features, such as sample size limitations and outcomes selected (e.g., systolic blood pressure), these studies are unable to offer clinically meaningful evidence of an effect of prayer that is as conclusive as the results of the Byrd study.

A study recently published in the *Western Journal of Medicine* by researchers at the California Pacific Medical Center addressed the limitations of earlier research. This double-blind, randomized, controlled trial investigated what it termed "distant healing" as a treatment in 40 volunteer AIDS patients with advanced cases of disease. Patients were randomly assigned to treatment and control groups; treatment was for one hour a day, six days a week, for ten weeks. All patients received standard medical care throughout the study.

Investigators recruited forty distant healers from eight traditions, including Christians, Jews, Buddhists, Native Americans, students of shamanism, and graduates of training programs in bioenergetic and meditative healing. Healers averaged seventeen years of experience. They were assigned on a rotating basis, each patient receiving treatment from a different healer each week. The concept of distant healing was given its ultimate test: healers were scattered throughout North America. They had only the first name and photograph of their respective patients, whom they never met.

Results provide dramatic, clinically meaningful evidence of a healing effect of prayer in patients with a life-threatening chronic disease. A medical chart review—also conducted in blinded fashion—found that subjects, compared to controls, had acquired fewer new AIDS-related illnesses (0.1 vs. 0.6 average per patient); had less severe illness (severity scale score of 0.8 vs. 2.65); required fewer physician visits (9.2 vs. 13.0), fewer hospitalizations (0.15 vs. 0.6), and fewer days of hospitalization (0.5 vs. 3.4); and subjects had improved mood according to scores on the Profile of Mood States scale (–26 vs. 14).

What We Know, What We Don't Know

This research underscores an observation commonly made by scientists working in this field. Successful absent prayer or distant spiritual intercession has effects on healing that have little to do with the religious background or ideology of the pray-er or healer. In reviewing this body of research for his best-selling book *Healing Words*, Dr. Larry Dossey came to the same conclusion: "Practically anyone's prayers appeared effective, regardless of their religious persuasion. This implied that no denomination or religion has a monopoly on prayer."

Despite these observations, there is a lot we still do not know about how prayer heals. I would second the conclusion of Dr. Michael E. McCullough, who reflected on the limitations of this field. Writing in the *Journal of Psychology and Theology* in a review of scientific studies of both intercessory prayer and prayer used as a coping device, he noted, "At this time, research on prayer and health is relatively primitive." Carefully controlled human investigations such as the Byrd and California Pacific studies are exceptions. But their results are useful guideposts, pointing to where we need to follow up. These studies offer confirmation that such phenomena are real.

Links in a Chain:
Prayer→Divine Intercession→Healing

In an interesting article published in the *Journal of Religion and Health*, psychologists Dr. Paul N. Duckro and Dr. Philip R. Magaletta of Saint Louis University reviewed evidence linking prayer to health and healing. They concluded, as did Drs. Mc-Cullough, Dossey, and Benor, that despite design limitations, studies on this question suggest a real connection. While not offering conclusive proof, the research makes a good case for absent prayer. If nothing else, this work, especially the Byrd and California Pacific studies, should alert scientists that something here is worth examining further.

Duckro and Magaletta go on to make a very important point: "Demonstrating positive outcomes of prayer is not equivalent to unmasking the mechanism by which the effects of prayer are accomplished. Studies hoping to do so necessarily enter much trickier waters."

The resistance and hostility that some scientists and physicians show to this topic stem, I believe, from an unwillingness to consider explanations that undermine a strictly materialistic worldview. These often involve concepts like God, spirit, divine mind, faith in Jesus Christ, higher consciousness, subtle energies, and the paranormal. Surprisingly, the mainstream biomedical establishment was not always so squeamish.

JAMA Acknowledges Religion, Sort Of

In 1997, I was solicited by *JAMA*, official journal of the American Medical Association, to briefly review published research linking religion and spirituality to health. This included both epidemiologic studies and experimental trials of prayer. When the article was published in *JAMA* and I received my copy of the journal, I was shocked to discover that parts of my final manuscript had been excised. It had been done without my prior knowledge, without consulting me or allowing me to see page proofs of the article. This type of behavior on the part of a peer-reviewed journal or its editor is almost unheard of in academic circles. What had they removed, and why?

I had begun my paper by citing a three-part series of articles on the topic of religious healing that had been published in *JAMA* over seventy years earlier. My point, obviously, was that the idea that prayer, faith, and spiritual intercession are capable of healing illness was not new. Further, the possibility had been taken very seriously and deemed worthy of investigation and comment by the American Medical Association long before any of the current editors were born.

The series, called "Religious Healing: A Preliminary Report," was written by Dr. Alice E. Paulsen under the auspices of the Committee on Public Health Relations of the New York Academy of Medicine. Dr. Paulsen surveyed the history and activities of healing prayer–oriented movements, such as Christian Science, Jewish Science, Divine Science, New Thought, Spiritualism, and Theosophy, as well as efforts of Protestant and Catholic churches. She considered many possible explanations for the apparent successes of these groups' efforts at healing: psychosomatic factors, hypnosis, suggestion, mental states, emotional effects, personality, religious faith, a subtle energy flow, and the presence of an omnipotent God.

Dr. Paulsen's list of possible explanations was as thorough as any proposed today. She acknowledged that some of her proposals were unusual and challenged current biomedical knowledge. (They still do today.) But this should not be an impediment, she asserted, to their proper investigation: "It may well be that religious healing makes use of forces not ordinarily recognized. It remains for us to study the nature of these forces, to determine how far they are present in the normal person, how far they may be applied with sanity, and what method of application is most advantageous."

These are hardly reckless comments. The problem, then as now, seems to be that some speculation is considered beyond the pale, and cannot be allowed to be broached. Investigating the mechanisms that might explain certain observable phenomena that have yet to be understood is part of what it means to do science. But when it comes to absent prayer or spiritually based healing, some men of science in Dr. Paulsen's day felt otherwise. As she noted, "The medical profession has largely ignored and even denied the possibility of this method of approach."

If anything, the situation is worse today. At least three-quarters of a century ago, *JAMA* allowed Dr. Paulsen's ideas to be published. Today, these same ideas apparently cannot be cited in an article.

How Prayer Heals

Much has been written lately in the press about research on prayer and healing, but the nuances of what these findings mean have gotten lost in the translation. This has resulted in distortions that promote overly simplistic images of God and the supernatural. It also has reinforced unrealistic expectations of how prayer might operate as a force for good in human affairs.

In 1997, I published my own take in the journal *Alternative Therapies*. In my article, "How Prayer Heals," I suggested several reasonable explanations for the positive results observed in studies of prayer and healing. Where these explanations differ from each other has to do with two key issues: first, the manner in which the healing effects of prayer operate or manifest in space and time; and second, the origin or source of healing in response to prayer.

How Healing Is Transmitted from Healer to Healee

A fundamental distinction can be made between healing that can, and healing that cannot, be explained by a universe that has what physicists call "local" characteristics. According to traditional, Newtonian physics, our universe is entirely local. That is, it consists of objects separated by space and time, and it operates according to certain mechanistic laws—for example, the inverse-square rule, whereby force dissipates as it distances itself from its origin. Space is three-dimensional and time is linear. In these terms, noncontact healing is understandable if we hypothesize, for example, that the

healing effects of prayer are due to subtle energies that are trans-
ferred along a pathway from a pray-er who is physically near the
pray-ee. But what about absent prayer?

Concepts of space and time as local present intractable problems for understanding the healing effects of absent prayer. No subtle energy yet identified has been shown to maintain its healing
power over vast distances or times—not in a way that can account
for the results of the Byrd or California Pacific studies. For these
experiments to have worked, something else must have been taking
place that was not caused by a physical energy as we know it and
that violates the assumption that the universe is entirely local. The
results of these experiments make sense, however, if the physical
universe has "nonlocal" characteristics.

According to physicists, as I described in my *Alternative Therapies* article, "the statistical predictions of quantum mechanics are
not fully explainable by the local universe believed in by most Western scientists and physicians, but instead require a nonlocal universe in which events or observations, regardless of their spatial
separation, can be 'correlated,' or influence each other instanta-
neously."

The concept of nonlocality was first fleshed out by physicist Dr.
David Bohm as he struggled to voice his dissatisfactions with quantum theory. He felt that the prevailing view of a universe frag-
mented into objects separated by space and time was false. He
introduced to physics the idea that the physical universe is characterized by an intrinsic wholeness and interconnectedness. In *The
Holographic Universe*, the late Michael Talbot explained the implications of Bohm's perspective for our understanding of space and
place: "At the level of our everyday lives things have very specific
locations, but Bohm's interpretation of quantum physics indicated
that at the subquantum level, the level in which the quantum potential operated, location ceased to exist. All points in space became
equal to all other points in space, and it was meaningless to speak of
anything as being separate from anything else."

Theoretical and experimental work by physicists Dr. John S.
Bell and Dr. Alain Aspect, among others, proves that nonlocality is

not just a concept debated by scientists, but is real. Separateness of individual objects in space and time is apparently an illusion. This amounts to asserting "that there is no here and there or that here is identical to there." If that is true, as best-selling author Gary Zukav has noted, "then we live in a nonlocal universe...characterized by superluminal (faster than light) connections between apparently 'separate parts.'"

Nonlocal Mind and "Physics Envy"

While nonlocality is fast becoming old news to a generation of physicists, biomedical science has not yet caught on. This is ironic. Medicine, according to Dr. Larry Dossey, suffers acutely from what he termed "physics envy." In a review of his book *Beyond Illness*, I elaborated on his idea: "Dossey describes this as a reliance upon a reductionistic, materialistic approach apparently founded on hard science, on the atomistic truths of physics. The irony is that allopathic medicine is not even being true to its own envy; the physics to which it clings has been outdated for most of the twentieth century."

Dr. Dossey's great contribution has been his effort to reconcile medicine with new developments in physics, such as nonlocality. He is also responsible for extending discussion of nonlocality to matters of human consciousness. In *Recovering the Soul*, he introduced the concept of "nonlocal mind"—the idea that nonlocality is characteristic not just of the physical universe but of our minds. He described the implications:

> If the mind is nonlocal in space and time, our interaction with each other seems a foregone conclusion. Nonlocal minds are *merging* minds, since they are not "things" that can be walled off and confined to moments in time or point-positions in space.
>
> If nonlocal mind is a reality, the world becomes a place of interaction and connection, not one of isolation and disjunction.

The implications for our understanding of all sorts of unusual transpersonal phenomena—absent prayer, psychic abilities, healing at a distance, intuitive connections between twins and spouses—are obvious. Because of nonlocal mind, much of the hypothetically "superempirical" may really be empirical. So many phenomena may be perceived as controversial and unproved only because skeptical physicians, psychologists, and scientists have failed to acknowledge discoveries made by physicists decades ago.

In his classic book *The Roots of Consciousness*, researcher Dr. Jeffrey Mishlove has summed up the question nicely: "The confirmation of this principle of *nonlocality* suggests that psi phenomena, if they exist, need not be in conflict with the established laws of science."

In other words, the idea that prayer at a distance is capable of healing is not as far-out as one might imagine. At least it is not ruled out by any inherent laws of physics that render it impossible. If current views of physicists are taken into account, the therapeutic efficacy of healing prayer is both possible and probable.

Natural versus Supernatural

As for the source of answered prayers, there are also two possibilities. Hypothetically, the healing response to petitionary prayer may originate from within nature—the observable physical universe—or partly or entirely from outside of nature. Explanations for the healing power of prayer based on the former assumption are what I have termed "naturalistic." Those based on the latter assumption I have called "supernatural."

Most prevailing explanations for how prayer heals are naturalistic. They do not imply or require the existence of God or a divine being who has supernatural characteristics—who is transcendent, or "located" at least in part outside of nature. Naturalistic explanations for how prayer heals are typically based on scientifically verifiable concepts—observable phenomena known to biology or physics. The "links in the chain" described in the first five chapters of this book, for example—behavior, social relationships, emotions, beliefs, thoughts—are all naturalistic explanations for how religion affects health. Similar explanations have been proposed for the healing effects of prayer.

In a discussion in *Advances*, journal of the Fetzer Institute, I proposed naturalistic explanations for the results of many of the existing studies of prayer and healing. None of these hypothetical explanations invokes concepts that are particularly controversial. They are all decidedly exoteric.

> For example, experiencing the presence of a healer or healers may foster a sense of belonging or support, which research shows is healthful. Being the object of prayer or of laying on of hands or other ritualized activity may stimulate an endocrine or immune response facilitative of healing. The physical preparations for healing (for example, preliminary fasts, meditation, abstentions of one sort or another) may themselves be promotive of health. Finally, expectations of healing—regardless of the real efficacy of the healer, for esoteric or exoteric reasons—can lead to physical changes.

These explanations work fine, but only in certain circumstances. When pray-er and pray-ee are in close proximity or are the same person, or when the pray-ee is aware that others are praying, these possibilities offer the most parsimonious explanations for how prayer heals. But instances of absent healing, where the recipient of prayer is blinded from the intervention, require something more. It is difficult to attribute results of the Byrd or California Pacific studies, for example, to the positive expectations of experimental subjects since those patients were not even aware that they *were* experimental subjects.

Several other explanations for the results of studies of absent prayer have also been proposed, such as the "superempirical" variety described in Chapter 6. Commentators on the growing body of prayer and healing studies have invoked many unusual concepts as potential explanations, using terms such as "paraphysical" or "magnetic," "extended mind," "morphic fields," "nonlocal mind," "transpersonal," "psi," and "consciousness." To these I could add "subtle energies," "altered states," and other terms derived from parapsychology.

Such concepts are controversial. Some scientists believe that they are real; others are more skeptical. There is no consensus among scientists as to whether superempirical phenomena exist or are worth studying. But if they are real, they are intrinsically naturalistic. The fact that these phenomena may seem to "violate the tenets of prevailing biomedical conceptions of physical law," as I noted in *Alternative Therapies*, may be due more to our gaps in knowledge about the nature of the universe than to their transcendence of the laws of physics. Such laws, by definition, cannot be breached. Perhaps our current knowledge is limited. The laws of the universe that most of us learned in school have failed to keep up with the developments of modern physics, as noted in the discussion of nonlocality.

By contrast, an entirely different possibility exists for the reason that some people heal after they are prayed for by others: they are healed because God or a divine being that hears and responds to prayers chooses to heal them. Because such a being resides fully or partly in a realm that transcends, or is outside of, the natural universe that it created, its actions are termed "supernatural." As I have noted:

> While not a universal conception of the deity, such a perspective is a cornerstone of many of the world's faith traditions. Indeed, the possibility that there is a Creator-God who volitionally chooses to answer or not answer petitionary prayers by means which entirely transcend any naturalistic mechanism may be the most commonly held belief of people who use prayer or spiritual interventions for friends or loved ones who are ill.

This is not to say that God or a higher power cannot also heal through the natural laws of the universe. Many devout religious believers acknowledge the hand of God in "normal" healing, such as through the natural biological and psychological processes of the human body. Others see in healing by means of superempirical mechanisms, such as a subtle bioenergy, the presence of God's loving grace. After all, according to this perspective, these energies and forces were engineered by the Creator for salutary purposes. Notwithstanding these other possibilities, healing through supernatural intercession represents a category of explanation for the healing effects of prayer that, true or not, is distinct from naturalistic theories.

Science Confronts the Supernatural

This hypothetical explanation for why prayer heals cannot easily be accommodated by science, scientists, or scientific methods. As I have explained:

> The idea that there is such a Being as this who exists and operates outside of the natural universe—locally, nonlocally, or however— may be a challenging notion to rational scientists and physicians. Moreover, if such supernatural healing does occur, it cannot be "proved" by studies ground in the research methods of naturalistic science; it must be taken on faith.... [S]cientific methods based on observation of natural phenomena cannot be used to verify processes that are purported to exist, in principle, outside of nature.

Science, by definition, will never be able prove the existence of supernatural healing. No research study that we could possibly ever conduct is capable of demonstrating that a partly or fully transcendent divine being responds positively to prayer by circumventing the natural laws that it created. But the same naturalistic research methods of science that cannot be used to prove the existence of the supernatural likewise cannot disprove it.

In the acknowledgments section of his published study in the *Southern Medical Journal*, Dr. Byrd stated, "I thank God for responding to the many prayers made on behalf of the patients." This was a sweet gesture, even if it can never be verified that Dr. Byrd's subjects got better because of something that God did. It could be that healing was attributable to a subtle energy unknowingly projected from healers to healees, or to the nonlocal effects of the healers' loving conscious intent, or to some other force, energy, power, or law that while unusual or currently unknown is nonetheless part of the natural order of things. Or it could be that Dr. Byrd is right: the Judeo-

Christian God answers the prayers of believers, as promised in the Jewish and Christian scriptures (Proverbs 15:29; Matthew 18:19-20).

Lessons to Consider

The evidence in this chapter gives rise to our seventh principle of theosomatic medicine:

PRINCIPLE 7

Absent prayer for others is capable of healing by paranormal means or by divine intervention.

What can we learn from findings linking absent prayer or spiritual intercession to physical and psychological healing? Is there evidence to conclude that religion affects our health across the natural history of disease? That is, as a force both for prevention of morbidity and mortality in healthy people *and* for healing of disease in people who are ill? Does a clear consensus exist as to how and why prayer leads to healing?

As we have seen in the preceding chapters, there is overwhelming evidence that practicing religion and being religious or spiritual are epidemiologically protective factors. Notwithstanding the usual caveats—that the findings express associations that exist on average and across populations—we can safely say that religion and health are connected in many ways. On the whole, this relationship seems to be a positive one. Valid and statistically significant associations have been observed in many different populations and settings. Numerous "links in the chain" have been proposed that can account for such associations in terms that are acceptable to mainstream biomedical science.

The evidence linking prayer to healing in humans, in my opinion, is less conclusive. Excellent controlled studies in human subjects, such as the Byrd and California Pacific experiments, are the exception. While I find their results convincing, the current state of experimental research on prayer and healing in humans suffers in comparison to research on the epidemiology of religion. Work in the latter field, as we have seen, rests on a foundation of hundreds of studies conducted in every imaginable geographical location and population group over a period of many decades. This is not to suggest that there are no naysayers—just that lack of replication is the last thing for which anyone could fault this field. The same cannot yet be said for research on prayer and healing.

Another important factor limiting widespread acceptance of these results is the lack of clear consensus about how absent prayer heals. Some scientists and physicians refuse to accept the results of entirely sound experiments that seem to implicate unusual mechanisms of action. Dr. Larry Dossey has collected some of the more hilarious closed-minded responses of scientists to studies that implicate superempirical mechanisms. My favorite, from a peer-reviewer for a scientific journal: "This is the kind of thing that I would not believe even if it existed."

Questions to Reflect On

This chapter began with my own story of healing. Facing the week-long marathon of my Ph.D. exams—an exhaustive ordeal in an otherwise healthy person—I had a fluke accident that left me in incredible pain with broken ribs and two nonfunctional arms. With nowhere else to turn, I sought the prayers of others. Apparently, they worked. What should have been a six-week recovery period was telescoped down to a day and a half.

My experience of being healed by the prayers of others had a lasting effect on me. Not just on my ribs and elbows, to be sure, but on my appreciation of how limited our current knowledge is when it comes to those factors that science says can possibly affect our health. According to the consensus of most biomedical scientists, I would imagine, what happened to me is impossible. Or at least it is due to other more mundane factors unrelated to absent prayer, such as misdiagnosis or my own positive expectations (although I am waiting for someone to tell me how expectations in someone asleep or passed out can completely heal broken bones overnight).

I have no doubt about what happened. Many people prayed, and I got better. Whatever the mechanism, I believe that it had little to do with the power of positive thinking or other factors intrinsic to my own local mind.

What happened to me is not unique. Far from it. Whenever I speak at conferences or tell this story to colleagues, I am met with many similar stories in return. Almost everyone, it seems, either knows someone who has reported such a healing or has experienced something like it themselves. What causes a particular person to heal in response to the prayers of others may have to remain a mystery. Is it the grace of a loving God? An unusual although naturalistic force or energy? Nonlocal connections among the consciousnesses of all people? Something else?

Epidemiology can only educate us as to generalized associations—for example, between smoking and lung cancer—and is unable to explain cases of disease in individual people. So, too, are the theories offered to account for the observed link between prayer and healing incapable of determining how or why any given person responds to prayer. That is to be worked out between a person and his or her God. The questions that follow can help us to do just that—to sort out what we believe about prayer, the presence of miracles, and the possibility of divine or supernatural healing.

1. Have you ever offered intercessory prayer to God for the healing of others? If you do not believe in a personal God, have you ever directed love, energy, spirit, or consciousness to another person for purposes of physical or emotional healing? Have you ever been the recipient of such prayers or intentionality? Have you ever prayed for another's healing without the other person's knowledge? If you were in need of healing, would you want others to pray for you even if they were unable to check with you first? Do you pray for healing differently from the way you usually pray? More intensely? More often? More humbly? Do you ever pray from within a state of meditation?

2. Do you believe in miracles—in the occurrence of blessings that defy the known laws of physics or nature? Do you believe that there is a God or a higher power that responds to people's

prayers for healing? Do you believe that this can happen through supernatural means? Or does God only answer prayers indirectly—such as through guiding the hands of physicians? Can we guarantee that God answers our prayers for healing affirmatively? Are there things we do that interfere with our prayers being answered? Are there some people whom God will not heal? How do you know? Do you believe that active faith or belief in God is a necessary condition of divine healing? Or can the prayers of others be answered even if the recipient does not believe or is unconscious? Does God have a hand in all physical healings, even those that result from normal medical treatment and where no prayer is offered up? Can all healing be thought of as a miracle?

3. Have you ever received what you believe to be a miraculous or divine healing of some kind? Did this follow absent prayers offered up by others? Did this follow some other type of distant intentionality on the part of others (e.g., meditation, visualization, sending energy or love)? Did you, or they, prepare in some way to petition God, such as through praise or worship or meditation or fasting? Do you believe that this had a role in the prayers being answered? Have you ever prayed for another person who was subsequently healed? Have you ever offered up prayers for another who then was not healed? Was there a difference in the way you prayed? If not, why do you believe one was healed and the other not? Could it have had something to do with the feelings you had for them personally? Something else entirely? Why do you think God or an ultimate loving force chooses to heal people or make them whole? Do you think that sometimes God chooses not to do so?

From Body-Mind to Body-Mind-Spirit

When it comes to health and well-being, research shows that how we express ourselves spiritually definitely matters. Whom we affiliate with, how often we participate with others, whether we make time for regular devotion, what we believe, the strength of our faith, experiences we have—these things contribute to whether we become ill or stay well.

To illustrate this, in *God, Faith, and Health* I have described results of scientific studies that underscore the health effects of religion in the lives of ordinary people. I also have described what I believe to be the future of medicine and biomedical science. These two things are very much related.

Models of Health, Healing, and Medicine

A new perspective is rapidly emerging on why we become sick, why we get better, and how we can remain healthy. It is notable for including a much wider range of factors than previously were considered to be determinants of health.

Physicians and epidemiologists long have known that certain physical factors are causally related to health. These include heredity and family history, the environment, and physiological and biological processes. This was Western medicine's dominant, and mostly exclusive, perspective until about forty years ago.

Since then, another set of factors—scientists call them "psychosocial"—has been found to be as important as physical factors for health and healing. These include healthy behavior, social relationships, positive emotions, personality traits and psychological characteristics, and healthy beliefs and attitudes; all have been described in this book. Recognition that physical factors act in conjunction with psychosocial factors has caused a sea change in how physicians and scientists view the body, define health, and practice medicine. The change is profound, and its implications have not escaped the attention of visionary thinkers in medicine who consider them signs of a significant paradigm shift.

In his brilliant book *Recovering the Soul,* Dr. Larry Dossey, for example, proposed that modern scientific medicine has passed through two eras or time periods. Era I, "materialistic medicine," was characterized by a machinelike view of humans as nothing but a body—a sack of bones swishing about in a soup of chemicals. Our bodies were believed to function according to strict laws, whereby health and disease occurred only as a result of physical processes. Era II, "mind-body medicine," began with the influx of psychosomatic and behavioral research and therapies that acknowledge the effects of our thoughts, feelings, and behavior on health and healing. Innovations such as behavior change programs, psychotherapy, biofeedback, and psychoneuroimmunology are examples of clinical advances since the emergence of this second era of scientific medicine.

The Era II perspective, however, is not the final one. Evidence presented here suggests something fundamentally different from, and beyond, body-mind medicine. In a future Era III, Dr. Dossey contends, physicians and scientists will come to accept evidence that "minds are spread through space and time; are omnipresent, infinite, and immortal; and are ultimately one."

This sounds a lot like how mystics, theologians, and religious scholars describe God, a divine presence, ultimate reality, the soul, or our higher spiritual self. *According to the scientific evidence presented in this book, this new era of medicine is no longer hypothetical.* Research findings suggest that we are on the verge of a medical revolution— yet another paradigm shift. The emerging medical model postulates that body, mind, and something beyond mind—call it "spirit"—work together to promote health, prevent illness, and produce healing.

Toward a Theosomatic Medical Model

Scientific evidence of links among body, mind, and spirit challenge our assumptions about what it means to be human, how we become sick, and how we can attain health. The body-mind, or psychosomatic, approach begins with a more realistic sense of what it means to be a human being than does the body-only perspective, to be sure. But the body-mind approach, like the body-only approach, does not go far enough. Evidence presented here suggests that there is something more to attaining health than just good genes or the right attitude. That "something" cannot be accounted for even by the best psychosocial theories or the principles of behavioral medicine. It has to do with engaging in spiritual pursuits and deepening our relationship with God or the eternal, with our own higher self, and with fellow participants in the spiritual quest.

I have termed this new perspective that acknowledges the spiritual determinants of health "theosomatic medicine." This phrase means, literally, a view of the determinants of health based on the apparent connections between God or spirit—or faith in God—and the well-being of the body. These precise connections are spelled out in the seven principles of theosomatic medicine that I have introduced in this book.

This perspective surely presents obvious challenges for those stuck in the body-only era of medicine. It also may be challenging even for those who are willing to accept body-mind principles but are unwilling to go further. Several years ago, in a scholarly article written with my colleague Dr. Harold Y. Vanderpool, I noted that "Western biomedicine...is still wrestling with a body-mind dualism that defies consensus; thus...any resolution of a body-mind-spirit pluralism is simply beyond consideration."

The assumptions of the body-as-machine perspective still hold sway in most medical specialties. This is evidenced by the continued attraction of costly, high-tech diagnostic and therapeutic procedures.

The cutting edge of research, to medical scientists, remains an Era I vision: more powerful drugs; more sophisticated surgical techniques involving lasers, bionics, and implantation; and more intricate genetic manipulation. The body-mind revolution might never have happened, for all that Western medicine seems to notice or care. This is a tragedy, because an even more profound revolution looms on the medical horizon. A lot of scientists and physicians do not "get it," and they risk being left behind, just like those doctors of the last century who persisted in bleeding their patients or conducting examinations or surgery without first washing their hands. As usual, Dr. Dossey has summarized things most concisely: "To omit the spiritual element from our medical worldview is not only narrow and arbitrary, it appears increasingly to be bad science as well."

The Triune Nature of Human Beings

One barrier, above all others, impedes acceptance that body, mind, and spirit work together for health. This barrier is a worldview that excludes soul or spirit or something transcendent from what it means to be human. If one believes that we have only a physical nature—that we are nothing but bodies—it is unlikely that any amount of scientific evidence on body-mind connections will be persuasive of the relevance of research in psychosomatic and behavioral medicine. Some proponents of the body-only view pay lip service to the idea of mind, but only as an epiphenomenon of neurochemistry and biological processes. This may sound like body-mind talk, but it is not.

Likewise, if we are body and mind, joined together—but no more—the idea of theosomatic medicine makes little sense. Just as some scientists feign interest in body-mind issues but rely on explanations based on physiology, other scientists profess to acknowledge the human spirit but tend to equate it with the psyche. Accordingly, whether we are bodies only, or bodies and minds, no part of us is eternal or touches the transcendent—which itself is an imaginary concept. This may sound like body-mind-spirit talk, but it is not.

Western biomedicine is cautious about acknowledging that there is a spiritual dimension to human life. Other religious and healing systems throughout the world are not as reticent. The idea that each human being is a nexus of body, mind, and spirit is present in numerous traditions.

The theologies and cosmologies of Western and Eastern spiritual paths alike endorse the idea that humans are triune in nature. The word "triune" means "three in one," and is often used in connection with the Christian concept of the trinity—the union of Father, Son, and Holy Spirit in one godhead. In the context of human nature, the word "triune" has a different meaning: that every human life incorporates physical, mental and emotional, and spiritual components. How these components are described, and how they are believed to interrelate, naturally differ across religions. But the three components—body, mind, and spirit—are present in some form.

Likewise, many systems or philosophies of healing operate under the assumption of a triune human nature. Unlike allopathic biomedicine—the dominant Western philosophy of medicine—ancient systems of healing typically operate from the presumption that humans comprise body, mind, and spirit. Their theories of disease causation and healing, their modes of history-taking and diagnosis, and their methods of treatment differ accordingly from allopathic models and procedures, which limit their focus primarily to the physical body. Such systems prove that theosomatic medicine is not such a new idea after all.

The principle underlying theosomatic medicine is that of a triune human nature—the idea that human life consists of distinct physical, mental and emotional, and spiritual dimensions. Triunity, in one form or another, is present in many religious and spiritual traditions. It is also at the core of many folk or alternative systems of medicine and healing. Let us look at a few examples.

Triunity in Yoga

In the yoga philosophy, a distinction is made among three types of disciplines, or pathways to self-actualization. The three paths to union (yoga) with the divine emphasize three separate domains of life that draw on and strengthen different aspects of personhood—body, mind, and spirit.

The disciplines of *karma* yoga, *jñana* yoga, and *bhakti* yoga represent the paths of action, learning, and devotion, respectively. Implicit in this three-part distinction is acknowledgment of our triune nature—we have bodies that engage in physical behavior, minds that engage in thinking, and something like a spirit or soul that can relate to God or the eternal through worship. Each of these dimensions of our nature can be used for secular or holy concerns. The advanced yogi, or master, will strive to engage all parts of his or her nature in service to the divine: asceticism and hard work to purify the body, study of sacred teachings to gain knowledge, and "complete surrender to the will and grace of God," as the late Dr. Heinrich Zimmer put it. Together these actions of body, mind, and spirit transform life into a sacred ritual.

More than a decade ago, I took part in a ten-day silent retreat at a yogic ashram. This spiritual community, located in western Virginia in the Appalachian foothills, was a beautiful and spiritually inspiring place. While there, I got a taste of the daily life of the permanent residents. Each day, residents and visitors took part in activities designed to make use of body, mind, and spirit for purposes of community building and worshiping the divine.

Mornings began with *pranayama* and *hatha* yoga—ritual breathing exercises and physical postures, respectively. Throughout the day, there were assigned periods of labor. Permanent residents had regular tasks; visitors like me were given one-hour assignments. One day I helped terrace a garden. Another day I licked envelopes. I also recall smashing boulders and carrying rocks as part of a landscaping crew. Residents called this physically demanding and exhausting labor "doing *karma* yoga."

Other times were set aside for formal learning. Our retreat schedule included individual and group study of sacred religious teachings—the Gita, the Upanishads, and writings of spiritual masters. Since it was a silent retreat, we could not ask questions, but I recall the experience as being very mentally stimulating. This engagement of the intellect gave participants a taste of the *jñana* path.

Finally, every morning, afternoon, and evening, there were special times for individual and community devotion. This included meditation, prayer, and silent contemplation. On the weekend, special programs were scheduled with music, chanting, and *darshan* (audience) with the leader of the community. I am sure that as a visitor and a Jew, I did not attach the same meaning to these experiences as did other participants and residents who might have been on a yogic spiritual path. But I, too, had a palpable sense of being in the presence of the sacred as all of us gathered to perform *bhakti* yoga—to connect with and worship God—in our own ways.

Triunity in Christian Theology

The distinction among body, mind, and spirit is not unique to the yogic tradition. Nor is the recognition of balance among these human dimensions as being central to a full and mature spiritual life. These same tenets are integral to the systematic theology of theologian Paul Tillich, a key figure in twentieth-century Christianity. In his classic *Dynamics of Faith*, Tillich outlined a model of faith as a balance of physical, intellectual, and devotional action.

According to Tillich, faith can be defined as "ultimate concern." Being ultimately concerned involves a centered act of the whole person directed toward something or someone transcendent. What qualifies as transcendent differs for different people. It may be "the Mosaic law, or Jesus as the Christ, Mohammed the prophet, or Buddha the illuminated." Regardless, to truly express our faith in the transcendent, we must marshal all of our resources—all parts of our nature. The most complete and mature expression of religious faith requires equal parts will, intellect or reason, and emotion. The absence or overabundance of any one or these elements represents a distortion of faith.

Tillich described how faith requires our physical action (in the form of behavior), our mental action (in the form of reasoning and thinking), and our affective action (in the form of feelings and emotions directed toward God). Through a balanced effort of all three types of human action—involving body, mind, and spirit—we can tap into something "unconditional," "infinite," and "ultimate" that is greater than the sum of the parts. When we do this, we become aware of the holy, which Tillich defined as awareness of the presence of the divine. This is mysterious and transcendent and, Tillich asserted, "It precedes, accompanies and follows all...activities of healing."

Triunity in Theosophy

Another version of our triune nature is found within esoteric traditions such as Theosophy. This philosophical system offers "divine truth" about God, humans, and the universe, described in works such as *The Secret Doctrine*. Theosophical teachings are strikingly similar to beliefs espoused by devotees of the esoteric paths of the world's established religions. So similar, in fact, despite dramatic differences in outward expression, that scholars speak of how their inner or core aspects converge along a common path. This "perennial philosophy," as it is often called, has also been referred to as the "primordial tradition," "secret wisdom," "forgotten truth," "ancient theology," and "ageless wisdom."

In Theosophy, as in other mystical traditions, human beings are said to consist of several overlapping, interpenetrating bodies or sheaths. These include the physical and etheric bodies; the astral and mental bodies; and the causal and higher bodies. These bodies vary in the denseness or subtlety of their energetic vibration, and each represents the manifestation of a human being in a particular plane or dimension.

The physical body is our three-dimensional physical vehicle—the visible part of us that sees, hears, tastes, smells, and feels. The etheric body is sometimes called the "aura." It is an invisible sheath that conforms to the template of our physical body. Some healers and intuitives claim to be able to see or otherwise perceive it.

The astral and mental bodies, respectively, are home to our emotions and thoughts. People who report out-of-body experiences often state that they are aware of being in a sort of body made of light, able to pass through solid matter. The building blocks of this dimension—the "things" one encounters—are said to consist of feelings and "thought-forms" rather than the solid objects of our physical world.

The causal body, in this perspective, is subtler still. It is home to the unique higher self that is eternal, "the receptacle of all that is enduring." This goes by various names—"soul," "ego," "monad"—and is the spark of the divine that incarnates as a whole person, gathering about it each of the successively denser bodies.

Theosophy's distinctions among subtler and denser manifestations of human energy clearly adhere to a triune view of human nature. The physical and etheric, astral and mental, and causal sheaths correspond to what is elsewhere termed "body," "mind," and "spirit" or "soul." Theosophical teachings on this matter may be unfamiliar or seem unusual from the perspective of traditional religion. The differentiation of physical, mental/emotional, and spiritual bodies, however, is a near universal teaching of esoteric and mystical schools and philosophies, varying only in terminology.

Triunity in Native American Medicine

The triune nature of human beings is an implicit feature of many systems and philosophies of medicine and healing. In the Native American medical tradition, according to author and shaman Ken "Bear Hawk" Cohen, physical, mental, and spiritual factors influence definitions of health, taxonomies of disease, and the practice of healing. To be a healthy person and to live a healthy life require maintaining a state of balance and harmony, keeping good thoughts, and directing gratefulness and respect to the creation and the Creator.

"Health and disease," Cohen has noted, "always have both physical and spiritual components....Health means restoring the body, mind, and spirit to balance and wholeness." The idea of wholeness is integral to Native American conceptions of human life and human well-being. According to Cohen, this tradition holds that all things are connected and "part of a single whole which is greater than the sum of its parts," namely, the Great Spirit, or God. A spiritual element, tied up with physical and mental or emotional determinants, is significant for all illnesses. It must be accounted for in diagnosis and addressed in treatment.

Triunity in Hebraic Medicine

These perspectives on the presence and unity of body, mind, and spirit are similar in many respects to those espoused by what Dr. Gerald Epstein, a well-known New York psychiatrist and author, has called "Hebraic medicine."

In his studies of comparative religion and alternative medicine, Dr. Epstein noticed that many religious traditions have developed a corresponding system of healing at some point in their history. The Hindu and yogic traditions produced Ayurvedic medicine; from Tibetan Buddhism came Tibetan medicine; traditional Chinese medicine grew from the spiritual heritage of China; and the Unani medical system has flourished in the Muslim world of South Asia. Esoteric philosophies, too, have developed corresponding systems of healing, notably Anthroposophical medicine and the teachings of Edgar Cayce. In each tradition, spiritual teachings and medical wisdom go hand in hand. The latter is intrinsically related to the former, and distinctions between "religious" and "medical" knowledge are often impossible to make. The idea of spirit or soul is as central to etiology and therapy as it is to spirituality.

Dr. Epstein wondered if Judaism, too, had evolved a system of medicine and healing. To his great delight, he discovered that it had. Dr. Epstein identified and described a "Western spiritual medical tradition," grounded in the teachings of the Torah, *Tanakh* (Bible), Talmud, and other Jewish sacred writings, that is as coherent and fleshed-out as any other religiously based healing system. One encyclopedic compendium of medical knowledge gleaned from Jewish scriptures, Dr. Julius Preuss's *Biblical and Talmudic Medicine*, reads like a comprehensive medical textbook, its six hundred-plus pages filled with details on anatomy, physiology, pathology, and treatment for every bodily system.

After surveying this material, as well as the healing-related insights of Jewish mystics, Dr. Epstein identified key features of the Hebraic medical tradition. Central to this philosophy is the "bodymind unity," by which is meant the inseparability of body and mind. Each is so bound up in the other that one cannot even speak of cause and effect when mapping their interconnection.

For illness to be healed, the natural processes of the bodymind must operate. This in turn "requires a degree of faith on the patient's part," and the most effective way to evoke such faith is by "[r]emembering God." In this way physical, mental or emotional, and spiritual factors work in tandem to promote health and well-being.

How the Theosomatic Model Is Changing Medical Practice

The idea that each human being consists of body, mind, and spirit is not new. Our triune nature is a fundamental premise of systems of religion and healing throughout the world. But a theosomatic medical model is not central to Western scientific medicine. Despite research evidence such as the studies summarized in this book, the view that something akin to the human spirit or faith in God has something to do with our health has been viewed as little more than superstition or, at best, as a nuisance to be accommodated.

Material on the epidemiologic and clinical significance of religion typically has not been included in predoctoral and post doctoral medical education. Biomedical professionals typically believe that humans are carnal bodies and nothing more. Physicians rarely inquire about the spiritual life of their patients, despite evidence of its importance for health and psychological well-being. Medical researchers, clinicians, and educators who continue to ignore this information do so at their own peril.

These long-standing trends suddenly are changing. More and more, medical practitioners, teachers, and scientists are coming to realize that findings such as the ones summarized here signal that they must start changing how they do things.

The fourth edition of the American Psychiatric Association's authoritative *Diagnostic and Statistical Manual of Mental Disorders*, known as DSM-IV, now includes a category describing disruptions in one's religious or spiritual life as a source of psychological distress. The new diagnostic category represents an official acknowledgment that issues such as religious conversion, changes in levels of religious commitment, and loss or questioning of faith or other spiritual values can have deleterious effects on well-being. This development has historical importance for medicine.

Some experts believe that the new DSM category is just the first step to wider acceptance of the idea that intense spiritual episodes—including mystical and near-death experiences, spiritual emergence, results of meditation, the loss of a spiritual teacher, and religious practice during terminal illness and in overcoming addiction—have life-changing consequences. According to the developers of this new diagnostic category:

> In the face of psychiatry's long-standing tendency either to ignore or pathologize the religious and spiritual dimensions of human existence, the inclusion of a religious or spiritual problem in the DSM-IV marks a significant breakthrough. For the first time, there is an acknowledgment of psychological problems of a religious or spiritual nature that are not attributable to a mental disorder.... [This] new diagnostic category could help to promote a new relationship between psychiatry and the fields of religion and spirituality that will benefit both mental health professionals and those who seek their assistance.

How the Theosomatic Model Is Changing Medical Education

At the same time, medical educators have begun to recognize that the training of compassionate and sensitive clinicians requires a focus on the spiritual needs of patients. Developing medical school courses on the topic of religion and spirituality has not been easy. Many academic scientists and clinicians consider it a "soft" subject that has no place in evidence-based medical education. Research in the epidemiology of religion is key to changing attitudes among those who have the authority to redirect how physicians are trained. Scientific studies such as those my colleagues and I have conducted have already had considerable impact on medical school deans and educators. Things are progressing very quickly.

Over the past few years, the John Templeton Foundation has provided grant funding to nearly two dozen medical schools for the purpose of adding educational content on the topic of spirituality. An equal number of medical schools already include courses, electives, rotations, or lectures on religious and spiritual issues. In all, about a third of U.S. medical schools now address faith and spirituality in their curricula. About a hundred medical schools have applied to Templeton for funding. The products of this new wave of medical education will be the first generation of physicians trained under a theosomatic model.

In a review published in *Academic Medicine*, the official journal of the Association of American Medical Colleges, Drs. Christina M. Puchalski and David B. Larson of the National Institute for Healthcare Research described the core features of this new approach to medical education. While different schools approach the topic of spirituality in different ways, common elements can be identified. These include (1) teaching spiritual assessment as part of taking a routine history, (2) reviewing scientific findings on the epidemiology of religion, (3) using case reports to illustrate the potentially harmful effects of religious beliefs, (4) instructing how to communicate more effectively with chronically ill and dying patients, (5) providing skills needed to break bad news in a compassionate manner, (6) summarizing health-related beliefs and practices of major religious traditions, and (7) helping medical students to explore their own spiritual perspectives for the purpose of greater self-awareness.

How the Theosomatic Model Is Changing Medical Research

Both the U.S. government and private foundations have sponsored major conferences and comprehensive summaries of existing research on the epidemiology of religion. Medical practitioners, educators, and scientists now have little excuse for ignoring the health effects of religious practice, spirituality, and faith in God. The old complaints that "no one's ever looked at that" and that "there's no evidence that that's true" no longer hold water.

Since the mid-1990s, the National Institutes of Health has convened expert panels to look into religion and health. Several NIH branches, including the National Institute on Aging, the Office for Behavioral and Social Sciences Research, and the National Center for Complementary and Alternative Medicine, have sponsored conferences or issued requests for research proposals in this area. As a result, scientists at North American universities, medical and nursing schools, and schools of public health are developing studies of the health-promoting, disease-preventing, and healing effects of religious and spiritual involvement. A growing number of these studies are being funded by the NIH.

Private foundations have followed suit. The Templeton Foundation published a two-hundred-page consensus report, *Scientific Research on Spirituality and Health*, summarizing existing studies. The National Institute for Healthcare Research published an outstanding research summary called *The Forgotten Factor in Physical and Mental Health*. This report consists of several modules and has been used in seminars and short courses. The John E. Fetzer Institute, a funding source for much of the pioneering work in body-mind medicine, has begun to support research on connections among body, mind, and spirit. A recent Fetzer Institute publication, developed in conjunction with the NIH, provides a useful summary of existing measures of religiousness and spirituality. This report will be invaluable to researchers and clinicians who want to assess these phenomena in a reliable and meaningful way.

The support of both the NIH and private foundations has enabled several universities to establish research centers on religion and health. Foremost among these is Duke University's Center for the Study of Religion/Spirituality and Health, under the direction of Dr. Harold G. Koenig, the leading clinical researcher in this field. Dr. Koenig is conducting numerous ongoing studies and trials. He has especially focused on the role of religion in recovery from illness.

These new studies build nicely on the mostly epidemiologic research, described in this book, on the preventive effects of religion for subsequent illness. Faith in God not only is epidemiologically significant, as we have seen, but may be therapeutically significant as well. This theme is taken up in Dr. Koenig's book, *The Healing Power of Faith*. The role of faith and spirituality as means of coping with existing physical or mental illness, and potentially hastening a cure, is an exciting frontier that physician-researchers are beginning to explore.

The Theosomatic Model and the Future of Medicine

The research findings summarized in this book herald a new era in medicine and biomedical science—a post psychosomatic era. Studies in the epidemiology of religion, coupled with the results of experimental trials of prayer and spiritual intercession, signal that the "biopsychosocial" perspective on health and healing does not go far enough.

Articulated in the 1970s by Dr. George L. Engel and others, this model of the social and psychological determinants of health and illness was an influential antidote to the reductionism of the prevailing body-only model. The body-mind orientation did a lot of good. It broadened the perspectives of two generations of medical practitioners and researchers. It signaled that people were tired of a mechanistic view of human beings, and all that it implied in the way of impersonal, technologically oriented medical care. It expanded concepts of what matters for health and healing to a wider range of personal characteristics—relationships, behaviors, attitudes, emotions, beliefs, thoughts, and values.

For all the good accomplished, body-mind medicine is not so much the ultimate "new paradigm" that so many have hoped for as it is a transitionary phase in the process of change to a more comprehensive model. By acknowledging that spirit matters—that the spiritual lives of human beings have health-promoting, disease-preventing, and therapeutic consequences—the theosomatic approach promises a real revolution in biomedical science, and ultimately, in medical care.

I believe that as the new theosomatic medical model gains acceptance, it will spell the end, once and for all, of the dominance of the mechanistic approach to defining human beings, promoting health, and healing illness. In my opinion, Western medicine is terminal. When the end comes near, changes will be swift and profound.

I believe that the body-only model of what it means to be a human, as well as sole reliance on the slash-and-drug model of therapy, is outdated and will soon fade from the scene. Lots of practitioners operating within that model do not know this, and when things collapse it will hit them unaware. Some defenders of the orthodox view, however, do know that the day is coming, and they are struggling to stay in control. Like many organisms right before they die, the current system is thrashing and rattling about; but it will not be long.

The purely psychosomatic, body-mind model of the determinants of health and healing will also be supplanted. The theosomatic perspective will become the standard approach to epidemiology, biomedical science, and the healing arts sometime in the twenty-first century. If we could float above the linear time flow of history and look down at the past couple of centuries and the new century, this would all be apparent. The twentieth-century allopathic biomedical model, as it has existed in the West since the early 1900s, will have been just a brief interlude that emerged as a corrective for the last time the pendulum swung too far in the other direction, in less rational times.

The Coming Medical Revolution

In 1995, Dr. Richard L. Garrison of the Department of Family Medicine at Baylor wrote a brilliant article, "The Five Generations of American Medical Revolutions," published in the *Journal of Family Practice*. His thesis was that all revolutions—whether political, like the American Revolution, or scientific, like the rise of Western biomedicine—follow discernible stages that correspond to generational groupings.

According to Dr. Garrison, the first stage is characterized by an inspirational call to arms involving a small group of people. The second stage sees synthesis of a comprehensive agenda. In the third stage, opportunists hop on board, the movement begins to become co-opted, and to use a sociological term, things become "routinized." By the fourth stage, the original spark that lit the revolution is long gone, and things become institutionalized and bureaucratized, with power centralized in a cabal. Finally, the fifth stage sees the oligarchy turn to reactionary means to hold on to their power, as the whole model degenerates and collapses. Those still clinging to power become the repressors of the first and second generation of visionaries of the succeeding revolution, which is by then already under way.

It is not hard to see that we are late in stage five of the current biomedical model. This model is materialistic, grounded in the view that human beings are physical bodies and nothing more. It is mechanistic and reductionistic—dominated by superspecialized practitioners who use high technology to zero in on and fix narrowly defined functional problems. Moreover, it is not even under the control of practitioners. Those days are long gone. Western scientific medicine is dominated by administrators trained to focus on the bottom line, instead of the well-being of people. This is equally true of the medical care establishment and the scientific research establishment.

As a result of this orientation—materialistic, mechanistic, reductionistic, financially driven—catastrophic mistakes are made every day. They are rarely acknowledged, though they often result in a loss of human lives. There are clinical errors—such as treatments selected on the basis of cost rather than need. There are also scientific errors—such as research studies that fail to assess factors that we now know significantly affect health and healing—such as religious involvement, spirituality, and faith and belief in God or a higher power.

This model is about to give up the ghost, and Dr. Garrison is blunt in his assessment: "Many authors say that we are surrounded by revolutionary changes in health care. On the contrary, I propose that we are mired in reactionary suppression of revolutionary ideas. I further propose that the frantic resistance to change is a sign that the present medical care system is growing weak and will soon collapse."

The coming of the new model of medicine, which Dr. Garrison says will be a generalist model, is inevitable: "The time for attempting to repair the present medical system has passed.... It is time for that paradigm to gracefully bow out, but I predict it will not do so. Those in influential positions will seek to preserve their advantages until forced from power."

How will this happen? As a scientist, I admit that I still cling to the idea that good science eventually drives out bad and that new ideas eventually replace outdated ones, even if it takes an awfully long time. As we have seen, good science is accumulating in droves, suggesting that the body-only and body-mind models of the determinants of health and healing are incomplete. The public is becoming aware of the new research and is demanding that practitioners pay attention. As we have witnessed with the expanding popularity of alternative therapies, if folks are not provided with what they want, they will vote with their feet, the current model will continue to lose market share, and that will be that.

I believe that the new generalist perspective, which is on the rise, will be based on something akin to a "unified field theory" of the determinants of health and healing. This perspective will not be grounded principally in genetics and molecular biology, as the mainstream medical research establishment presumes. Instead, it will be founded on an integrated, body-mind-spirit perspective—a view of all sentient life as part of a continuous bioenergetic spectrum, or to use a metaphor borrowed from author Ken Wilber, a "spectrum of consciousness." This will be the next era or historical epoch of Western medicine.

Throughout history, new medical and scientific discoveries have challenged existing worldviews, speeding up their reform or demise. The scientific findings presented in *God, Faith, and Health* dramatically broaden our perspective on what determines health. This new perspective promises nothing less than to accelerate the demise of a biomedical worldview that no longer has all the answers.

According to the theosomatic perspective, everything in existence—inside and outside of our bodies, from the smallest molecule to the actions of a loving God—is fair game for research on how and why people stay well, become ill, and get better. We ought to exclude nothing at all from our consideration. To do so without first having pursued a program of scientific investigation and come up empty-handed is to engage in what skeptics like to call "pseudo-science." With respect to the epidemiology of religion, a principal scientific foundation of the theosomatic model, we are hardly coming up empty. The weight of published evidence overwhelmingly confirms that our spiritual life influences our health. This can no longer be ignored.

References

1   ***One had the intriguing if innocuous title***   Thomas W. Graham, Berton H. Kaplan, Joan C. Cornoni-Huntley, Sherman A. James, Caroline Becker, Curtis G. Hames, and Siegfried Heyden (1978). "Frequency of Church Attendance and Blood Pressure Elevation." *Journal of Behavioral Medicine* 1: 37–43.

2   ***"A consistent pattern of lower systolic and diastolic"***   Ibid., p. 37.
    Fascinated, I read the next article   Berton H. Kaplan (1976). "A Note on Religious Beliefs and Coronary Heart Disease." *Journal of the South Carolina Medical Association* 15 (5, supplement): 60–64.
    "So we are left with a challenge to refine our concepts"   Ibid., p. 64.

4   ***In all, over half of U.S. medical schools***   Christina M. Puchalski and David B. Larson (1998). "Developing Curricula in Spirituality and Medicine." *Academic Medicine* 73: 970–974.
    In its September 3 issue, it published   Jeffrey S. Levin, David B. Larson, and Christina M. Puchalski (1997). "Religion and Spirituality in Medicine: Research and Education." *Journal of the American Medical Association* 278: 792–793.

6   ***In 1987, I published an article summarizing these results***   Jeffrey S. Levin and Preston L. Schiller (1987). "Is There a Religious Factor in Health?" *Journal of Religion and Health* 26: 9–36.

9   ***"While medical professionals have been"***   David B. Larson (1995). "Have Faith: Religion Can Heal Mental Ills." *Insight* (March 6) : 18–20.
    matters of "ultimate concern"   Paul Tillich (1957). *Dynamics of Faith*. New York: Harper and Row.

20   ***National surveys repeatedly show***   Andrew M. Greeley (1989). "Denominations." *Religious Change in America*. Cambridge, Mass.: Harvard University Press; pp. 21–41.
    In Dimensions of the Sacred   Ninian Smart (1996). "Doctrine, Philosophy and Some Dimensions." *Dimensions of the Sacred: Anatomy of the World's Beliefs*. Berkeley: University of California Press; pp. 27–69.

21   ***Most religions or denominations***   Leo Rosten (ed.) (1975). "Religious Beliefs and Credos—in Question-and-Answer Form." Part 1 in *Religions of America: Ferment and Faith in an Age of Crisis*. New York: Simon and Schuster; pp. 23-305.
    Jewish tradition, by contrast   Rabbi Yisrael Meir haKohen (The Chafetz Chayim) (compiler) (1990). *The Concise Book of Mitzvoth: The Commandments Which Can Be Observed Today*. Jerusalem: Feldheim Publishers.
    the soul transcends the need   Heinrich Zimmer (1951). "Upanisad." Part 3.3.2 in *Philosophies of India*. Bollingen Series, no. 26. Princeton, N.J.: Princeton University Press; pp. 355–378.
    In a review that my colleagues and I recently published   Jeffrey S. Levin, Linda M. Chatters, Christopher G. Ellison, and Robert Joseph Taylor (1996). "Religious Involvement, Health Outcomes, and Public Health Practice." *Current Issues in Public Health* 2: 220–225.

22   ***According to Dr. Rachel E. Spector***   Rachel E. Spector (1996). "Healing: Magicoreligious Traditions." *Cultural Diversity in Health and Illness*, 4th ed. Stamford, Conn.: Appleton and Lange; pp. 133–168.

24   *Scientists at the Missouri Center for Health Statistics*   Larry McEvoy and Garland Land (1981). "Life-Style and Death Patterns of the Missouri RLDS Church Members." *American Journal of Public Health* 71: 1350–1357.

        Investigators at the University of Colorado   Richard F. Hamman, Jerome I. Barancik, and Abraham M. Lilienfeld (1981). "Patterns of Mortality in the Old Order Amish: I. Background and Major Causes of Death." *American Journal of Epidemiology* 114: 845–861.

        A team from the University of Utah   Joseph L. Lyon, Harry P. Wetzler, John W. Gardner, Melville R. Klauber, and Roger R. Williams (1978). "Cardiovascular Mortality in Mormons and non-Mormons in Utah, 1969–71." *American Journal of Epidemiology* 108: 357–366.

        Researchers from the Institute for Social Medicine   J. Berkel and F. de Waard (1983). "Mortality Pattern and Life Expectancy of Seventh-Day Adventists in the Netherlands." *International Journal of Epidemiology* 12: 455–459.

        we felt a need existed to summarize these findings   Jeffrey S. Levin and Harold Y. Vanderpool (1989). "Is Religion Therapeutically Significant for Hypertension?" *Social Science and Medicine* 29: 69–78.

25   *including lower systolic and diastolic blood pressure*   Bruce Armstrong, Anthony J. Van Merwyk, and Harvey Coates (1977). "Blood Pressure in Seventh-Day Adventists." *American Journal of Epidemiology* 105: 444–449.

        In one Australian study   Ian W. Webster and Graeme K. Rawson (1979). "Health Status of Seventh-Day Adventists." *Medical Journal of Australia* 1: 417–420.

        A California study   Gordon R. Stavig, Amnon Igra, and Alvin R. Leonard (1984). "Hypertension among Asians and Pacific Islanders in California." *American Journal of Epidemiology* 119: 677–691.

        A famous study from the Harvard School of Public Health   Norman A. Scotch (1963). "Sociocultural Factors in the Epidemiology of Zulu Hypertension." *American Journal of Public Health* 53: 1205–1213.

        A follow-up study   Norman A. Scotch (1960). "A Preliminary Report on the Relation of Sociocultural Factors to Hypertension among the Zulu." *Annals of the New York Academy of Science* 84: 1000–1009.

        This is what Israeli researchers found   Y. Friedlander and J. D. Kark (1984). "Familial Aggregation of Blood Pressure in a Jewish Population Sample in Jerusalem Among Ethnic and Religious Groupings." *Social Biology* 31: 75–90.

26   *When researchers from the National Cancer Institute*   Frances B. Locke and Haitung King (1980). "Mortality among Baptist Clergymen." *Journal of Chronic Diseases* 33: 581–590.

        Japanese scientists conducted   Michiharu Ogata, Masato Ikeda, and Masanori Kuratsune (1984). "Mortality among Japanese Zen Priests." *Journal of Epidemiology and Community Health* 38: 161–166.

27   *Studies conducted at UCLA*   James E. Enstrom (1975). "Cancer Mortality among Mormons." *Cancer* 36: 825–841.

        George K. Jarvis (1977). "Mormon Mortality Rates in Canada." *Social Biology* 24: 294–302.

        Moreover, Mormons are protected   Joseph L. Lyon, Melville R. Klauber, John W. Gardner, and Charles R. Smart (1976). "Cancer Incidence in Mormons and Non-Mormons in Utah, 1966–1970." *New England Journal of Medicine* 294: 129–133.

        Joseph L. Lyon, John W. Gardner, Melville R. Klauber, and Charles R. Smart (1977). "Low Cancer Incidence and Mortality in Utah." *Cancer* 39: 2608–2618.

        Studies conducted at Loma Linda University   Roland L. Phillips, Lawrence Garfinkel, J. W. Kuzma, W. Lawrence Beeson, Terry Lotz, and Burton Brin (1980). "Mortality Among California Seventh-Day Adventists for Selected Cancer Sites." *Journal of the National Cancer Institute* 65: 1097–1107.

Roland L. Phillips, J. W. Kuzma, W. Lawrence Beeson, and Terry Lotz (1980). "Influence of Selection Versus Lifestyle on Risk of Fatal Cancer and Cardiovascular Disease among Seventh-Day Adventists." *American Journal of Epidemiology* 112: 296–314.

Frank R. Lemon, Richard T. Walden, and Robert W. Woods (1964). "Cancer of the Lung and Mouth in Seventh-Day Adventists." *Cancer* 17: 486–497.

Research from the prestigious Sloan-Kettering Institute Ernest L. Wynder, Frank R. Lemon, and Irwin J. Bross (1959). "Cancer and Coronary Artery Disease among Seventh-Day Adventists." *Cancer* 12: 1016–1028.

A study from the Danish Cancer Registry Ole Møller Jensen (1983). "Cancer Risk Among Danish Male Seventh-Day Adventists and Other Temperance Society Members." *Journal of the National Cancer Institute* 70: 1011–1014.

An Indiana University study Terrell W. Zollinger, Roland L. Phillips, and Jan W. Kuzma (1984). "Breast Cancer Survival Rates among Seventh-Day Adventists and Non-Seventh-Day Adventists." *American Journal of Epidemiology* 119: 503–509.

Scientists at Northwestern University Alice O. Martin, Judith K. Dunn, Joe L. Simpson, Carolyn L. Olsen, Sam Kemel, Michael Grace, Sherman Elias, Gloria E. Sarto, Blon Smalley, and Arthur G. Steinberg (1980). "Cancer Mortality in a Human Isolate." *Journal of the National Cancer Institute* 65: 1109–1113.

They also found advantages Alice O. Martin, Judith K. Dunn, and Blon Smalley (1980). "Use of a Genealogically Linked Data Base in the Analysis of Cancer in a Human Isolate." In *Cancer Incidence in Defined Populations*, edited by J. Cairns, J. L. Lyon, and M. Skolnick. Banbury Report 4. Cold Spring Harbor Laboratory: New York; pp. 235–255.

A study from the University of Alberta Kenneth Morgan, T. Mary Holmes, Michael Grace, Sam Kemel, and Diane Robson (1983). "Patterns of Cancer in Geographic and Endogamous Subdivisions of the Hutterite Brethren of Canada." *American Journal of Physical Anthropology* 62: 3–10.

28   *Dr. Benjamin Travers noted never having seen a case* Benjamin Travers (1837). "Observations on the Local Diseases Termed Malignant." *Medical and Chirurgical Transactions* 17: 337.

research showing an enormously higher Abraham L. Wolbarst (1932). "Circumcision and Penile Cancer." *The Lancet* 1: 150–153.

Much of this work was reviewed in 1948 E. L. Kennaway (1948). "The Racial and Social Incidence of Cancer of the Uterus." *British Journal of Cancer* 2: 177–212.

29   *A Dutch study from over 50 years ago* J. J. Versluys (1949). "Cancer and Occupation in the Netherlands." *British Journal of Cancer* 3: 161–185.

A study conducted at the University of Texas Medical Branch Bertram Herman and Philip E. Enterline (1970). "Lung Cancer among the Jews and Non-Jews of Pittsburgh, Pennsylvania, 1953–1967: Mortality Rates and Cigarette Smoking Behavior." *American Journal of Epidemiology* 91: 355–367.

Reviewing data sources from studies William Haenszel (1971). "Cancer Mortality among U.S. Jews." *Israeli Journal of Medical Science* 7: 1437–1450.

fewer respiratory symptoms Ernest L. Wynder, Frank R. Lemon, and Nathan Mantel (1965). "The Epidemiology of Persistent Cough." *American Review of Respiratory Diseases* 91: 679–700.

better cardiovascular health Webster and Rawson, op. cit.

less mortality Berkel and de Waard, op. cit.

higher life expectancy Frank R. Lemon and Jan W. Kuzma (1969). "A Biologic Cost of Smoking: Decreased Life Expectancy." *Archives of Environmental Health* 18: 950–955.

RLDS Mormons McEvoy and Land, op. cit.

Researchers have studied death rates Hamman, Barancik, and Lilienfeld, op. cit.

30   *Studies dating to the 1950s* Herbert Seidman, Lawrence Garfinkel, and Leonard Craig (1962). "Death Rates in New York City by Socio-Economic Class and Religious Group and by Country of Birth, 1949–1951." *Jewish Journal of Sociology* 1: 254–273.

In New York City, for example   David M. Liberson (1956). "Causes of Death among Jews in New York City in 1953." *Jewish Social Studies* 18: 83–117.

In a follow-up study of nearly 7,000 Californians   Deborah L. Wingard (1982). "The Sex Differential in Mortality Rates." *American Journal of Epidemiology* 115: 205–216.

Using data from the 1972–1977 General Social Survey   Lucy Y. Steinitz (1980). "Religiosity, Well-Being, and Weltanschauung Among the Elderly." *Journal for the Scientific Study of Religion* 19: 60–67.

In data from the 1984 General Social Survey   Kimberly Reed (1991). "Strength of Religious Affiliation and Life Satisfaction." *Sociological Analysis* 52: 205–210.

34   *Mormons are much less likely to smoke tobacco or drink alcohol*   John W. Gardner, Joseph L. Lyon, and Dee W. West (1984). "Cancer in Utah Mormons and Non-Mormons." *Journal of Collegium Aescuplapium* July: 15–24.

consume caffeinated beverages such as coffee or tea, or have multiple sexual partners D. W. West, J. L. Lyon, and J. W. Gardner (1980). "Cancer Risk Factors: An Analysis of Utah Mormons and Non-Mormons." *Journal of the National Cancer Institute* 65: 1083–1095.

Seventh-Day Adventists are more likely   Roland L. Phillips (1975). "Role of Life-style and Dietary Habits in Risk of Cancer among Seventh-Day Adventists." *Cancer Research* 35: 3513–3522.

Adventists who are stricter in their observance of dietary guidelines   Roland L. Phillips, Frank R. Lemon, W. Lawrence Beeson, and Jan W. Kuzma (1978). "Coronary Heart Disease Mortality among Seventh-Day Adventists with Differing Dietary Habits: A Preliminary Report." *American Journal of Clinical Nutrition* 31: S191–S198.

The Amish and Hutterites   Henry Troyer (1988). "Review of Cancer among 4 Religious Sects: Evidence that Life-Styles Are Distinctive Sets of Risk Factors." *Social Science and Medicine* 26: 1007–1017.

35   *"It appears that religious beliefs"*   Kenneth Vaux (1976). "Religion and Health." *Preventive Medicine* 5: 522–536; esp. p. 522.

These are the exact same behaviors identified as the most important targets   Department of Health and Human Services (1980). *Promoting Health, Preventing Disease: Objectives for the Nation*. Washington, D.C.: U.S. Government Printing Office.

These include the following activities   Vaux, op. cit.

Examples include less frequent use of mouthwash   Ernest L. Wynder, Geoffrey Kabat, Saul Rosenberg, and Marcia Levenstein (1983). "Oral Cancer and Mouthwash Use." *Journal of the National Cancer Institute* 70: 255–260.

36   *more frequent preventive medical behavior*   Edward Suchman (1964). "Sociomedical Variations among Ethnic Groups." *American Journal of Sociology* 70: 319–331.

greater likelihood of having received a diagnostic X-ray   Abraham M. Lilienfeld (1959). "Diagnostic and Therapeutic X-Radiation in an Urban Population." *Public Health Reports* 74: 29–35.

visiting a physician, taking medications, and staying home when ill   David Mechanic (1963). "Religion, Religiosity, and Illness Behavior." *Human Organization* 22: 202–208.

we summarized results of over thirty such studies   Preston L. Schiller and Jeffrey S. Levin (1988). "Is There a Religious Factor in Health Care Utilization?: A Review." *Social Science and Medicine* 27: 1369–1379.

This material was published in 1977 as a popular book   John H. Knowles (ed.) (1977). *Doing Better and Feeling Worse: Health in the U.S.* New York: W.W. Norton.

In "The Responsibility of the Individual," Dr. Knowles described   John H. Knowles (1977). "The Responsibility of the Individual." In *Doing Better and Feeling Worse: Health in the U.S.*, edited by John H. Knowles. New York: W.W. Norton; pp. 57–80.

37   *The greater importance during that period of advances in sanitation and hygiene* Thomas Mc-Keown (1979). *The Role of Medicine: Dream, Mirage, or Nemesis?* Princeton, N.J.: Princeton University Press.

"The individual has the power" Knowles, op. cit.

"50% percent of mortality" David A. Hamburg, Glen R. Elliott, and Delores L. Parron (eds.) (1982). *Health and Behavior: Frontiers of Research in the Biobehavioral Sciences.* Institute of Medicine publication no. 82-010. Washington, D.C.: National Academy Press.

constitute "behavioral pathogens" Joseph D. Matarazzo (1984). "Behavioral Immunogens and Pathogens in Health and Illness." In *Psychology and Health*, edited by Barbara L. Mammons and C. James Scheirer. Washington, D.C.: American Psychological Association; pp. 5–43.

38   *the famous "seven healthy practices"* Lisa F. Berkman and Lester Breslow (1983). *Health and Ways of Living: The Alameda County Study.* New York: Oxford University Press.

39   *One of the most interesting studies to come from the Alameda County data* Lisa F. Berkman and S. Leonard Syme (1979). "Social Networks, Host Resistance, and Mortality: A Nine-Year Follow-Up Study of Alameda County Residents." *American Journal of Epidemiology* 109: 186–204.

46   *Most Americans affiliate themselves with a religion* Andrew M. Greeley (1989). "Denominations." *Religious Change in America.* Cambridge, Mass.: Harvard University Press; pp. 21–41.

47   *These numbers have not changed much for decades* Andrew M. Greeley (1989). "Church Attendance." Chapter 4 in *Religious Change in America.* Cambridge, Mass.: Harvard University Press; pp. 42–56.

   Leo Rosten (ed.) (1975). "Church Attendance in the United States." *Religions of America: Ferment and Faith in an Age of Crisis.* New York: Simon and Schuster; pp. 431–436.

and may be declining somewhat Michael Hout and Andrew M. Greeley (1987). "The Center Doesn't Hold: Church Attendance in the United States, 1940–1984." *American Sociological Review* 52: 325–345.

One authoritative study compared people's reports of religious attendance C. Kirk Hadaway, Penny Long Marler, and Mark Chaves (1993). "What the Polls Don't Show: A Closer Look at U.S. Church Attendance." *American Sociological Review* 58: 741–752.

50   *our paper was published in* **Social Science and Medicine** Jeffrey S. Levin and Harold Y. Vanderpool (1987). "Is Frequent Religious Attendance *Really* Conducive to Better Health? Toward an Epidemiology of Religion." *Social Science and Medicine* 24: 589–600.

51   *more likely to rate their health as good* Jeffrey S. Levin and Kyriakos S. Markides (1986). "Religious Attendance and Subjective Health." *Journal for the Scientific Study of Religion* 25: 31–40.

report higher levels of well-being Jeffrey S. Levin and Kyriakos S. Markides (1988). "Religious Attendance and Psychological Well-Being in Middle-Aged and Older Mexican Americans." *Sociological Analysis* 49: 66–72.

experience less disability, fewer days in bed in the previous year, and fewer physical symptoms Jeffrey S. Levin and Kyriakos S. Markides (1985). "Religion and Health in Mexican Americans." *Journal of Religion and Health* 24: 60–69.

A Scottish study D. R. Hannay (1980). "Religion and Health." *Social Science and Medicine* 14A: 683–685.

Scientists from the University of Michigan James S. House, Cynthia Robbins, and Helen L. Metzner (1982). "The Association of Social Relationships and Activities with Mortality: Prospective Evidence from the Tecumseh Community Health Study." *American Journal of Epidemiology* 116: 123–140.

Scientists at Johns Hopkins University George W. Comstock and Kay B. Partridge (1965). "Church Attendance and Health." *Journal of Chronic Diseases* 25: 665–672.

A follow-up study found an actual **dose-response relationship** George W. Comstock and James A. Tonascia (1977). "Education and Mortality in Washington County, Maryland." *Journal of Health and Social Behavior* 18: 54–61.

52   *A study of churchgoers in Evans County, Georgia*   Victor J. Schoenbach, Berton H. Kaplan, Lisa Fredman, and David G. Kleinbaum (1986). "Social Ties and Mortality in Evans County, Georgia." *American Journal of Epidemiology* 123: 577–591.
      "epistemologically speaking"   Levin and Vanderpool, op. cit., pp. 590–591.

53   *Using data from the approximately 2,000 people interviewed*   Jeffrey S. Levin, Linda M. Chatters, and Robert Joseph Taylor (1995). "Religious Effects on Health Status and Life Satisfaction Among Black Americans." *Journal of Gerontology: Social Sciences* 50B: S154–S163.
      This scale summarized responses to questions   Jeffrey S. Levin, Robert Joseph Taylor, and Linda M. Chatters (1995). "A Multidimensional Measure of Religious Involvement for African Americans." *Sociological Quarterly* 36: 157–173.
            Linda M. Chatters, Jeffrey S. Levin, and Robert Joseph Taylor (1992). "Antecedents and Dimensions of Religious Involvement Among Older Black Adults." *Journal of Gerontology: Social Sciences* 47: S269–S278.
      religion tended to be downplayed or simply ignored   Jeffrey S. Levin and Sheldon S. Tobin (1995). "Religion and Psychological Well-Being." In *Aging, Spirituality, and Religion: A Handbook*, edited by Melvin A. Kimble, Susan H. McFadden, James W. Ellor, and James J. Seeber. Minneapolis, Minn.: Fortress Press; pp. 30–46.

54   *our article was one of only three studies to receive a perfect "10"*   Harold G. Koenig and Andrew Futterman (1995). "Religion and Health Outcomes: A Review and Synthesis of the Literature." Presented at the Conference on Methodological Approaches to the Study of Religion, Health, and Aging, National Institute on Aging, Bethesda, Md., March 16–17.
      We obtained data on nearly 6,000 adults   Jeffrey S. Levin and Linda M. Chatters (1998). "Religion, Health, and Psychological Well-Being in Older Adults: Findings from Three National Surveys." *Journal of Aging and Health* 10: 504–531.
      "replicated secondary data analysis"   Linda K. George and Richard Landerman (1984). "Health and Subjective Well-Being: A Replicated Secondary Data Analysis." *International Journal of Aging and Human Development* 19: 133–156.

55   *My colleague Dr. Ellison examined data*   Christopher G. Ellison (1995). "Race, Religious Involvement and Depressive Symptomatology in a Southeastern U.S. Community." *Social Science and Medicine* 40: 1561–1572.
      Religious attendance did even better   Jeffrey S. Levin, Kyriakos S. Markides, and Laura A. Ray (1996). "Religious Attendance and Psychological Well-Being in Mexican Americans: A Panel Analysis of Three-Generations Data." *The Gerontologist* 36: 454–463.

56   *presented an opportunity to replicate our findings*   Jeffrey S. Levin and Robert Joseph Taylor (1998). "Panel Analyses of Religious Involvement and Well-Being in African Americans: Contemporaneous vs. Longitudinal Effects." *Journal for the Scientific Study of Religion* 37: 695–709.
      Two of the most prominent psychosocial epidemiologists in the world   Ellen L. Idler and Stanislav V. Kasl (1997). "Religion Among Disabled and Nondisabled Persons II: Attendance at Religious Services as a Predictor of the Course of Disability." *Journal of Gerontology: Social Sciences* 52B: S306–S316.

57   *The best study conducted to date*   William J. Strawbridge, Richard D. Cohen, Sarah J. Shema, and George A. Kaplan (1997). "Frequent Attendance at Religious Services and Mortality over 28 Years." *American Journal of Public Health* 87: 957–961.

58   *Definitions abound*   Manuel Barrera Jr. (1986). "Distinctions Between Social Support Concepts, Measures, and Models." *American Journal of Community Psychology* 14: 413–445.
      emphasizing the structure and content of people's social networks and relationships   Kristina Orth-Gomér and Anna-Lena Undén (1987). "The Measurement of Social Support in Population Surveys." *Social Science and Medicine* 24: 83–94.

59   *A related distinction is often made*   Carma A. Heitzmann and Robert M. Kaplan (1988). "Assessment of Methods for Measuring Social Support." *Health Psychology* 7: 75–109.

Research over the past thirty to forty years Peggy A. Thoits (1982). "Conceptual, Methodological, and Theoretical Problems in Studying Social Support as a Buffer Against Life Stress." *Journal of Health and Social Behavior* 23: 145–159.

"individuals with a strong social support system" Ibid., p. 145.

In his presidential address to the American Psychosomatic Society Sidney Cobb (1976). "Social Support as a Moderator of Life Stress." *Psychosomatic Medicine* 38: 300–314.

"We have seen strong and often quite hard evidence" Ibid., p. 310.

60 *"information leading the subject to believe"* Ibid., p. 300.

he develops a model of the ways that religious involvement enables the receipt of social support Christopher G. Ellison (1994). "Religion, the Life Stress Paradigm, and the Study of Depression." In *Religion in Aging and Health: Theoretical Foundations and Methodological Frontiers*, edited by Jeffrey S. Levin. Thousand Oaks, Calif.: Sage Publications; pp. 78–121.

In Dr. Ellison's words Ibid., p. 79.

61 *Along with sociologist Dr. Linda K. George of Duke University* Christopher G. Ellison and Linda K. George (1994). "Religious Involvement, Social Ties, and Social Support in a Southeastern Community." *Journal of the Scientific Study of Religion* 33: 46–61.

By "informal support" they mean those types of assistance Robert Joseph Taylor, Irene Luckey, and Jacqueline Marie Smith (1990). "Delivering Services in Black Churches." In *The Church's Ministry with Families: A Practical Guide*, edited by Diana S. Richmond Garland and Diane L. Pancoast. Dallas: Word Publishing; pp. 194–209.

62 *More frequent church attendance* Robert Joseph Taylor and Linda M. Chatters (1986). "Church-based Informal Support Among Elderly Blacks." *The Gerontologist* 26: 637–642.

Among older adults, frequent church attendance Robert Joseph Taylor and Linda M. Chatters (1988). "Church Members as a Source of Informal Social Support." *Review of Religious Research* 30: 193–203.

Among the elderly Robert Joseph Taylor and Linda M. Chatters (1986). "Patterns of Informal Support to Elderly Black Adults: Family, Friends, and Church Members." *Social Work* 31: 432–438.

In 1988, a most unusual article appeared in Science James S. House, Karl R. Landis, and Debra Umberson (1988). "Social Relationships and Health." *Science* 241: 540–545.

The concept of social support long had been a principal focus of study Berton H. Kaplan, John C. Cassel, and Susan Gore (1977). "Social Support and Health." *Medical Care* 15 (5, supplement): 47–58.

63 *Their findings "manifest a consistent pattern of results"* House, Landis, and Umberson, op. cit., p. 542.

"More socially isolated or less socially integrated" Ibid., p. 540.

"The evidence on social relationships is probably" Ibid., p. 543.

"Social relationships have a predictive" Ibid., p. 544.

64 *a provocative article by scientists from Columbia University and UCLA* Bruce G. Link and Jo Phelan (1995). "Social Conditions as Fundamental Causes of Disease." *Journal of Health and Social Behavior* (extra issue): 80–94.

numerous outcomes, such as the onset of depression Charles J. Holahan and Rudolf H. Moos (1991). "Life Stressors, Personal and Social Resources, and Depression: A 4-Year Structural Model." *Journal of Abnormal Psychology* 100: 31–38.

recovery from heart disease and cancer Alan Reifman (1995). "Social Relationships, Recovery from Illness, and Survival: A Literature Review." *Annals of Behavioral Medicine* 17: 124–131.

self-ratings of overall health Frank W. Young and Nina Glasgow (1998). "Voluntary Social Participation and Health." *Research on Aging* 20: 339–362.

"The extent and quality of social relationships" House, Landis, and Umberson, op. cit., p. 544.

a theme that House had explored in a research study House, Robbins, and Metzner, op. cit.

In an article published in the **Journal for the Scientific Study of Religion** Levin and Markides (1986), op. cit., p. 32.

74 *"Consider your soul"* Sue Browder (1995). "Eight Easy Ways to Look—and Feel—Younger." *Reader's Digest* (September): 147–151.

the final key to "help you stay healthy" Ibid., p. 151.

75 *Data from the authoritative General Social Survey* Andrew M. Greeley (1989). "Devotions, Defections, Activities, and Attitudes." *Religious Change in America*. Cambridge, Mass.: Harvard University Press; pp. 57–66.

Sociologist Dr. Andrew M. Greeley notes Ibid.

We made several important observations Jeffrey S. Levin and Robert Joseph Taylor (1997). "Age Differences in Patterns and Correlates of the Frequency of Prayer." *The Gerontologist* 37: 75–88.

76 *According to a study by my colleagues* Christopher G. Ellison and Robert Joseph Taylor (1996). "Turning to Prayer: Social and Situational Antecedents of Religious Coping among African Americans." *Review of Religious Research* 38: 111–131.

77 *Participants in a study of more than 500 older Mexican Americans* Kyriakos S. Markides, Jeffrey S. Levin, and Laura A. Ray (1987). "Religion, Aging, and Life Satisfaction: An Eight-Year, Three-Wave Longitudinal Study." *The Gerontologist* 27: 660–665.

We replicated these findings Jeffrey S. Levin and Robert Joseph Taylor (1998). "Panel Analysis of Religious Involvement and Well-Being in African Americans: Contemporaneous vs. Longitudinal Effects." *Journal for the Scientific Study of Religion* 37: 695–709.

My colleague Dr. Ellison, along with his associates Christopher G. Ellison, David A. Gay, and Thomas A. Glass (1989). "Does Religious Commitment Contribute to Individual Life Satisfaction." *Social Forces* 68: 100–123.

78 *A provocative study examined effects of religious devotion* Marc A. Musick (1996). "Religion and Subjective Health Among Black and White Elders." *Journal of Health and Social Behavior* 37: 221–237.

which is commonly asked in epidemiologic studies Jeffrey S. Levin (1995). "Subjective Health, Screening, and Psychological Distress in African Americans." *Journal of Clinical Geropsychology* 1: 89–95.

one of the best predictors that we know of for mental health Linda K. George and Richard Landerman (1984). "Health and Subjective Well-Being: A Replicated Secondary Data Analysis." *International Journal of Aging and Human Development* 19: 133–156.

level of functional disability Erdman B. Palmore and Bruce M. Burchett (1997). "Predictors of Disability in the Final Year of Life." *Journal of Aging and Health* 9: 283–297.

rates of physician use Frederic D. Wolinsky and Rodney M. Coe (1984). "Physician and Hospital Utilization among Noninstitutionalized Elderly Adults: An Analysis of the Health Interview Survey." *Journal of Gerontology* 39: 334–341.

even longevity Ellen L. Idler and Yael Benyami (1997). "Self-Rated Health and Mortality: A Review of Twenty-seven Community Studies." *Journal of Health and Social Behavior* 38: 21–37.

79 *As with Dr. Ellison's findings for religious devotion and well-being* Ellison, Gay, and Glass, op. cit.

Another notable Duke study explored the impact of prayer Harold G. Koenig, James N. Kvale, and Carolyn Ferrel (1988). "Religion and Well-Being in Later Life." *The Gerontologist* 28: 18–28.

Drs. Musick and Koenig have since joined forces Marc A. Musick, Harold G. Koenig, Judith C. Hays, and Harvey Jay Cohen (1998). "Religious Activity and Depression Among Community-Dwelling Elderly Persons with Cancer: The Moderating Effect of Race." *Journal of Gerontology: Social Sciences* 53B: S218–S227.

81 *She was selected to write the chapter on religion and spirituality* Susan H. McFadden (1996). "Religion and Spirituality." In *Encyclopedia of Gerontology: Age, Aging, and the Aged*, vol. 2, edited by James E. Birren. San Diego, Calif.: Academic Press; pp. 387–397.

In our chapter in the **Handbook of Emotion, Adult Development, and Aging** Susan H. McFadden and Jeffrey S. Levin (1996). "Religion, Emotions, and Health." In *Handbook of Emotion, Adult Development, and Aging*, edited by Carol Magai and Susan H. McFadden. San Diego, Calif.: Academic Press; pp. 349–365.

This may be vital for elderly people struggling to "preserve the self" Sheldon S. Tobin (1991). "Preserving the Self Through Religion." *Personhood in Advanced Old Age: Implications for Practice*. New York: Springer Publishing Company; pp. 119–133.

82 *prayer can be divided into four categories* Margaret M. Poloma and George H. Gallup Jr. (1991). *Varieties of Prayer: A Survey Report*. Philadelphia: Trinity Press International.

"practicing the presence of God" Brother Lawrence (1985; original, 1692). *The Practice of the Presence of God*. Translated by Robert J. Edmonson; edited by Hal M. Helms. Orleans, Mass.: Paraclete Press.

"These types of prayer are not mutually exclusive" Levin and Taylor (1997), op. cit., p. 85.

seeking of an 'inward communion' William James (1958; original, 1902). *The Varieties of Religious Experience*. New York: Mentor; p. 352.

'into the presence of the ultimate mystery of God' Harry C. Meserve (1991). "The Human Side of Prayer." *Journal of Religion and Health* 30: 271–276.

Among observant Jews, for example Levin and Taylor, op. cit.

83 *In* **How I Pray,** *journalist Jim Castelli interviewed* Jim Castelli (ed.) (1994). *How I Pray*. New York: Ballantine Books.

"I've since grown out of that type of prayer" Ibid., pp. 137–138.

According to the late Dr. Joachim Wach Joachim Wach (1944). *Sociology of Religion*. Chicago: University of Chicago Press; p. 39.

84 *The nineteenth-century philosopher and psychologist Dr. William James* James, op. cit., pp. 76–139.

The most balanced type of religiousness Andrew R. Fuller (1994). "William James." *Psychology and Religion: Eight Points of View*, 3rd ed. Lanham, Md.: Littlefield Adams; pp. 1–33.

"I remembered having read" Norman Cousins (1979). *Anatomy of an Illness as Perceived by the Patient: Reflections on Healing and Regeneration*. Toronto: Bantam Books; pp. 34–35.

Hans Selye's classic book, **The Stress of Life** Hans Selye (1976). *The Stress of Life*, rev. ed. New York: McGraw-Hill.

85 *"It worked"* Cousins, op. cit., pp. 39–40.

"the will to live is not a theoretical abstraction" Ibid., p. 44.

86 *"The nerves are there, to be sure"* Ernest Lawrence Rossi (1993). *The Psychobiology of Mind-Body Healing: New Concepts of Therapeutic Hypnosis*, rev. ed. New York: W.W. Norton; pp. 133, 136.

These "messenger molecules" have also been called "molecules of emotion" Candace B. Pert (1998). *Molecules of Emotion: Why You Feel the Way You Feel*. New York: Scribner.

They comprise the neurotransmitters Rossi, op. cit., pp. 158–159.

Scientists have identified pathways between what are called "affective disturbances" Sheldon Cohen and Mario S. Rodriguez (1995). "Pathways Linking Affective Disturbances and Physical Disorders." *Health Psychology* 14: 374–380.

Emotions influence interactions Seymour Reichlin (1993). "Neuroendocrine-Immune Interactions." *New England Journal of Medicine* 329: 1246–1253.

modulate our immunity, up or down, with implications for disease Steven F. Maier, Linda R. Watkins, and Monika Fleshner (1994). "Psychoneuroimmunology: The Interface Between Behavior, Brain, and Immunity." *American Psychologist* 49: 1004–1017.

"the study of the psychological modulation" Ibid., p. 1009.

87   *These traps, which Dr. Borysenko called "the dirty tricks department of the mind"*   Joan
      Borysenko (1987). *Minding the Body, Mending the Mind.* Toronto: Bantam Books; p. 111.
      In so doing, we can develop healthier emotions   Ibid., pp. 34–36.
      In Opening Up, *Dr. Pennebaker explained*   James W. Pennebaker (1990). *Opening Up: The
      Healing Power of Confiding in Others.* New York: Avon Books.

88   *"It seems something deep inside our cells"*   Emrika Padus (1986). "Love." Chapter 69 in
      The Complete Guide to Your Emotions and Your Health: New Dimensions in Mind/Body Healing
      (pp. 647–648). Emmaus, Penn.: Rodale Press; p. 648.
      "Emotions impel us to express our feelings"   Leonard Laskow (1992). *Healing with Love:
      A Physician's Breakthrough Mind/Body Medical Guide for Healing Yourself and Others: The Art
      of Holoenergetic Healing.* San Francisco: HarperSanFrancisco; p. 43.
      "Unconditional love is the most powerful stimulant"   Bernie S. Siegel (1986). *Love, Med-
      icine and Miracles: Lessons Learned About Self-Healing from a Surgeon's Experience with Excep-
      tional Patients.* New York: Harper Perennial; p. 181.
      Through his Exceptional Cancer Patients (ECaP) program   Hal Morgenstern, George
      A. Gellert, Stephen D. Walter, Adrian M. Ostfeld, and Bernard S. Siegel (1984). *Journal of
      Chronic Diseases* 37: 273–282.

89   *to propose the "epidemiology of love" as a new scientific field*   Jeff Levin (2000). "A Pro-
      legomenon to an Epidemiology of Love: Theory, Measurement, and Health Outcomes."
      Journal of Social and Clinical Psychology 19: 117–136.
      "These positive affects may serve as sorts of psychic beta-blockers or emotional placebos"
      Jeffrey S. Levin and Harold Y. Vanderpool (1989). "Is Religion Therapeutically Significant
      for Hypertension?" *Social Science and Medicine* 29: 69–78; esp. p. 74.

90   *Dr. McCullough reviewed evidence that prayer may "facilitate improvements in mood"*
      Michael E. McCullough (1995). "Prayer and Health: Conceptual Issues, Research Review,
      and Research Agenda." *Journal of Psychology and Theology* 23: 15–29; esp. p. 17.

91   *worship marshals emotions that strengthen what epidemiologists call "host resistance"*
      Jeffrey S. Levin (1996). "How Religion Influences Morbidity and Health: Reflections on
      Natural History, Salutogenesis and Host Resistance." *Social Science and Medicine* 43:
      849–864.

93   *Duke University psychiatrist Dr. Harold G. Koenig*   Harold G. Koenig (1994). *Aging and
      God: Spiritual Pathways to Mental Health in Midlife and Later Years.* New York: The Haworth
      Press.

99   *Decades of research have shown*   Preston L. Schiller and Jeffrey S. Levin (1988). "Is
      There a Religious Factor in Health Care Utilization?: A Review." *Social Science and Medi-
      cine* 27: 1369–1379.

100   *later published in a peer-reviewed gerontology journal*   Jeffrey S. Levin (1997). "Reli-
      gious Research in Gerontology, 1980–1994: A Systematic Review." *Journal of Religious
      Gerontology* 10: 3–31.
      A retrospective study of 85 older Canadians   Bruce Hunsberger (1985). "Religion, Age,
      Life Satisfaction, and Perceived Sources of Religiousness: A Study of Older Persons." *Jour-
      nal of Gerontology* 40: 615–620.
      A nationally representative study   Lucy Y. Steinitz (1980). "Religiosity, Well-Being, and
      Weltanschauung Among the Elderly." *Journal for the Scientific Study of Religion* 19: 60–67.
      My colleague Dr. Christopher G. Ellison   Christopher G. Ellison (1991). "Religious
      Involvement and Subjective Well-Being." *Journal of Health and Social Behavior* 32:
      80–99.
      Scientists from Penn State University   Fern K. Willits and Donald M. Crider (1988).
      "Religion and Well-Being: Men and Women in the Middle Years." *Review of Religious Re-
      search* 29: 281–294.

101   *An extremely interesting study, conducted by a UCLA social scientist*   Marvin Pollner
      (1989). "Divine Relations, Social Relations, and Well-Being." *Journal of Health and Social
      Behavior* 30: 92–104.

A research team from the Vermont Regional Cancer Center   Jerome W. Yates, Bruce J. Chalmer, Paul St. James, Mark Follansbee, and F. Patrick McKegney (1981). "Religion in Patients with Advanced Cancer." *Medical and Pediatric Oncology* 9: 121–128.

102   *"may be at least as important as the more traditional psychological and secular social factors"*   Michael King, Peter Speck, and Angela Thomas (1994). "Spiritual and Religious Beliefs in Acute Illness—Is This a Feasible Area for Study?" *Social Science and Medicine* 38: 631–636; esp. p. 636.

103   *"obviously do not exhaust all of the basic religious tenets"*   Neal Krause (1993). "Measuring Religiosity in Later Life." *Research on Aging* 15: 170–197; esp. p. 195.
"beliefs that cut across specific faiths"   Ibid.
It has been suggested that specific religious beliefs   Lucille B. Bearon and Harold G. Koenig (1990). "Religious Cognitions and Use of Prayer in Health and Illness." *The Gerontologist* 30: 249–253.
"prayer and medical help-seeking are not mutually exclusive"   Ibid., p. 249.

104   *"religious beliefs are indeed intertwined"*   Ibid., p. 253.
In her outstanding textbook   Spector, op. cit., pp. 133–168.
In the first edition   Rachel E. Spector (1979). *Cultural Diversity in Health and Illness*. New York: Appleton and Lange; pp. 114–123.

105   *By the fourth edition*   Spector (1996), op. cit.
"dictates social, moral, and dietary practices"   Ibid., pp. 144–145.
spirituality is as much a dimension of health   Paul Tillich (1981; original, 1961). *The Meaning of Health*. Richmond, Calif.: North Atlantic Books; pp. 57–58.

107   *Dr. Kenneth A. Wallston, Vanderbilt psychology professor*   Kenneth A. Wallston, Barbara S. Wallston, and Robert DeVellis (1978). "Development of the Multidimensional Health Locus of Control (MHLC) Scales. *Health Education Monographs* 6: 160–170.
"style of living characterized by extremes"   C. David Jenkins (1971). "Psychologic and Social Precursors of Coronary Disease." *New England Journal of Medicine* 284: 244–255, 307–317.
In a famous essay published in 1904   Max Weber (1958; original, 1904–5). *The Protestant Ethic and the Spirit of Capitalism*. New York: Charles Scribner's Sons.

108   *may reflect "the cultural context of the Protestant ethic"*   Karen A. Matthews (1982). "Psychological Perspectives on the Type A Behavioral Pattern." *Psychological Bulletin* 91: 293–323; esp. p. 304.
"Central to the notion of Type A behavior"   Lewis H. Margolis, Kenneth R. McLeroy, Carol W. Runyan, and Berton H. Kaplan (1983). "Type A Behavior: An Ecological Approach." *Journal of Behavioral Medicine* 6: 245–258; esp. pp. 254–255.
"What part does this 'ethic' in fact play"   Berton H. Kaplan (1976). "A Note on Religious Beliefs and Coronary Heart Disease." *Journal of the South Carolina Medical Association* 15 (5, supplement): 60–64; esp. p. 63.
Recently, an interesting effort was made to test the possibility   Adrian Furnham (1990). "The Protestant Work Ethic and Type A Behaviour: A Pilot Study." *Psychological Reports* 66: 323–328.

109   *Using data from a well-known study of more than 400 air traffic controllers*   Jeffrey S. Levin, C. David Jenkins, and Robert M. Rose (1988). "Religion, Type A Behavior, and Health." *Journal of Religion and Health* 27: 267–278.

110   *Along with my colleague Dr. Preston L. Schiller*   Jeffrey S. Levin and Preston L. Schiller (1986). "Religion and the Multidimensional Health Locus of Control Scales." *Psychological Reports* 59: 26.
"a function of the relationship between religion and control"   Daniel McIntosh and Bernard Spilka (1990). "Religion and Physical Health: The Role of Personal Faith and Control Beliefs." In *Research in the Social Scientific Study of Religion: A Research Annual*, vol. 2, edited by Monty L. Lynn and David O. Moberg. Greenwich, Conn.: JAI Press; p. 169.

111 *Our health beliefs and the knowledge that we have about health* Judith Green and Robert Shellenberger (1991). "Self Regulation for Health." *The Dynamics of Health and Wellness: A Biopsychosocial Approach.* Fort Worth, Texas: Holt, Rinehart and Winston; pp. 315–350.

112 *"synthesize information from medical and psychiatric practice"* John J. Schwab (1985). "Psychosomatic Medicine: Its Past and Present." *Psychosomatics* 26: 583–593; esp. p. 588.
"the notions of mind and body refer to inseparable and mutually dependent aspects of man" Z. J. Lipowski (1984). "What Does the Word 'Psychosomatic' Really Mean? A Historical and Semantic Inquiry." *Psychosomatic Medicine* 46: 153–171; esp. p. 159.
"certain attributes of functions of the organism" Ibid., p. 162.
the interface of "personal characteristics and processes" C. David Jenkins (1985). "New Horizons for Psychosomatic Medicine." *Psychosomatic Medicine* 47: 3–25.

113 *just like cigarette smoking and high cholesterol* Meyer Friedman and Ray Rosenman (1974). *Type A Behavior and Your Heart.* Greenwich, Conn.: Fawcett Publications.
Two of these, anger and hostility Karen Matthews, David Glass, Ray Rosenman, and Rayman Bortner (1977). "Competitive Drive, Pattern A, and Coronary Heart Disease: A Further Analysis of Some Data from the Western Collaborative Group Study." *Journal of Chronic Diseases* 30: 489–498.
but it sparked considerable interest in anger and hostility Redford Williams (1989). *The Trusting Heart.* New York: Times Books.

114 *"The 'mind' that the concepts of Type A and hostility both presume"* Harris Dienstfrey (1991). "Type A and the Emotions That Can Lead to Heart Disease." *Where the Mind Meets the Body: Type A, the Relaxation Response, Psychoneuroimmunology, Biofeedback, Neuropeptides, Hypnosis, Imagery and the Search for the Mind's Effects on Physical Health.* New York: HarperPerennial; pp. 22–23.
Consider, for example, the findings Levin, Jenkins, and Rose, op. cit.
"With a concept like Type A" Dienstfrey, op. cit., p. 23.
personality factors "exert their impacts on health" Shelley E. Taylor (1990). "Health Psychology: The Science and the Field." *American Psychologist* 45: 40–50; esp. p. 42.

115 *Scientists from the University of Pittsburgh* Stanley H. King and Daniel H. Funkenstein (1957). "Religious Practice and Cardiovascular Reactions During Stress." *Journal of Abnormal and Social Psychology* 55: 135–137.
"given arithmetical problems to do in their heads" Ibid., p. 135.
reflected "a conception of God" Ibid., p. 136.

116 *Evidence from a study of nearly 400 Dutch adults* Johan Ormel, Roy Stewart, and Robert Sanderman (1989). "Personality as Modifier of the Life Change-Distress Relationship: A Longitudinal Modelling Approach." *Social Psychiatry and Psychiatric Epidemiology* 24: 187–195.
In their outstanding textbook Judith Green and Robert Shellenberger (1991). "Development of the Personality Characteristics of Healthy People." *The Dynamics of Health and Wellness: A Biopsychosocial Approach.* Fort Worth, Texas: Holt, Rinehart and Winston; pp. 559–590.
As defined by psychologist Dr. Suzanne Kobasa Suzanne Kobasa (1979). "Stressful Life Events, Personality and Health: An Inquiry into Hardiness." *Journal of Personality and Social Psychology* 37: 1–11.

117 *the degree to which one believes that one's life chances are under one's control* Leonard Pearlin and C. Schooler (1978). "The Structure of Coping." *Journal of Health and Social Behavior* 19: 2–21.
"the sum of evaluations across salient attributes" Jim Blascovich and Joseph Tomaka (1991). "Measures of Self-Esteem." In *Measures of Personality and Social Psychological Attitudes,* edited by John P. Robinson, Phillip R. Shaver, and Lawrence S. Wrightsman. San Diego: Academic Press; p. 115.

The most popular way to assess self-esteem   M. Rosenberg (1965). *Society and the Adolescent Self-Image*. Princeton, N.J.: Princeton University Press.

Among 500 middle-aged and older adults   Neal Krause and Thanh Van Tran (1989). "Stress and Religious Involvement Among Older Blacks." *Journal of Gerontology: Social Sciences* 44: S4–S13.

118   *Dr. Krause followed this up*   Neal Krause (1992). "Stress, Religiosity, and Psychological Well-Being Among Older Blacks." *Journal of Aging and Health* 4: 412–439.

A nationally representative Louis Harris survey   Neal Krause (1995). "Religiosity and Self-Esteem Among Older Adults." *Journal of Gerontology: Psychological Sciences* 50B: P236–P246.

119   *"Research that examines whether or not"*   Taylor, op. cit., p. 46.

each of these "special gifts and talents"   Berton H. Kaplan (1992). "Social Health and the Forgiving Heart: The Type B Story." *Journal of Behavioral Medicine* 15: 3–14; esp. p. 7.

120   *Religious beliefs enhance our "sense of intrinsic moral self-worth"*   Christopher G. Ellison and Jeffrey S. Levin (1998). "The Religion-Health Connection: Evidence, Theory, and Future Directions." *Health Education and Behavior* 25: 700–720; esp. p. 706.

we "construct personal relationships"   Ibid., p. 707.

"seem to be especially valuable in dealing with serious health problems"   Ibid.

"challenge fundamental premises of existence"   Ibid., pp. 707–708.

"reinforce basic role identities"   Ibid.

Research by the late Dr. L. Eugene Thomas   L. Eugene Thomas and Kim O. Chambers (1989). "Phenomenology of Life Satisfaction Among Elderly Men: Quantitative and Qualitative Views." *Psychology and Aging* 4: 284–289.

According to published studies   Ibid.

    L. Eugene Thomas (1992). "Identity, Ideology and Medicine: Health Attitudes and Behavior Among Hindu Religious Renunciates." *Social Science and Medicine* 34: 499–502.

127   *describing "the faith that heals"*   William Osler (1910). "The Faith That Heals." *British Medical Journal* (June 18): 470–472.

*Writing in the **Johns Hopkins Medical Journal***   Jerome D. Frank (1975). "The Faith That Heals." *The Johns Hopkins Medical Journal* 137: 127–131.

it serves to "mobilize the faith that heals"   Ibid., p. 129.

Dr. Matthews marshals evidence suggesting that expressions of faith   Dale M. Matthews (1998). *The Faith Factor: Proof of the Healing Power of Prayer*. New York: Viking.

128   *According to the late Dr. E. Mansell Pattison*   E. Mansell Pattison (1988). "Behavioral Psychology and Religion; A Cosmological Analysis." In *Behavior Therapy and Religion: Integrating Spiritual and Behavioral Approaches to Change*, edited by William R. Miller and John E. Martin. Newbury Park, Calif.: Sage Publications; pp. 171–186.

Utilizing the National Survey of Black Americans sample   Jeffrey S. Levin, Linda M. Chatters, and Robert Joseph Taylor (1995). "Religious Effects on Health Status and Life Satisfaction Among Black Americans." *Journal of Gerontology: Social Sciences* 50B: S154–S163.

129   *In this new study, we examined*   Jeffrey S. Levin and Robert Joseph Taylor (1998). "Panel Analyses of Religious Involvement and Well-Being in African Americans: Contemporaneous vs. Longitudinal Effects." *Journal for the Scientific Study of Religion* 37: 695–709.

In one study   Kyriakos S. Markides, Jeffrey S. Levin, and Laura A. Ray (1987). "Religion, Aging, and Life Satisfaction: An Eight-Year, Three-Wave Longitudinal Study." *The Gerontologist* 27: 660–665.

In another study   Jeffrey S. Levin and Kyriakos S. Markides (1985). "Religion and Health in Mexican Americans." *Journal of Religion and Health* 24: 60–69.

130   *Both groups are relatively homogeneous*   Andrew M. Greeley (1979). "Ethnic Variations in Religious Commitment." In *The Religious Dimension: New Directions in Quantitative Research*, edited by Robert Wuthnow. New York: Academic Press; pp. 113–134.

Using data from three large, nationally representative studies Jeffrey S. Levin and Linda M. Chatters (1998). "Religion, Health, and Psychological Well-Being in Older Adults: Findings from Three National Surveys." *Journal of Aging and Health* 10: 504–531.

Dr. Ellison and I are currently conducting another multisample study Jeffrey S. Levin and Christopher G. Ellison (1999). "Modeling Religious Effects on Health and Psychological Well-Being: A Replicated Secondary Data Analysis of Seven Study Samples." (Unpublished manuscript.)

131   *According to its developers at Harvard Medical School* Jared D. Kass, Richard Friedman, Jane Leserman, Patricia C. Zuttermeister, and Herbert Benson (1991). "Health Outcomes and a New Index of Spiritual Experience." *Journal for the Scientific Study of Religion* 30: 203–211.

including "a cognitive appraisal" Ibid., p. 204.

132   *A study using a random sample of more than 400 family practice patients* J. LeBron McBride, Gary Arthur, Robin Brooks, and Lloyd Pilkington (1998). "The Relationship Between a Patient's Spirituality and Health Experiences." *Family Medicine* 30: 122–126.

The original study that developed and validated the INSPIRIT Kass, Friedman, Leserman, Zuttermeister, and Benson, op. cit.

Researchers from Duke University David B. Larson, Harold G. Koenig, Berton H. Kaplan, Raymond S. Greenberg, Everett Logue, and Herman A. Tyroler (1989). "The Impact of Religion on Men's Blood Pressure." *Journal of Religion and Health* 28: 263–278.

133   *Scientists at Harvard and Yale* Diana M. Zuckerman, Stanislav V. Kasl, and Adrian M. Ostfeld (1984). "Psychosocial Predictors of Mortality among the Elderly Poor." *American Journal of Epidemiology* 119: 410–423.

134   *it is "unlikely that the benefits of religiousness"* Ibid., p. 417.

These results were confirmed in a clinical study at Dartmouth Thomas E. Oxman, Daniel H. Freeman Jr., and Eric D. Mannheimer (1995). "Lack of Social Participation or Religious Strength and Comfort as Risk Factors for Death After Cardiac Surgery in the Elderly." *Psychosomatic Medicine* 57: 5–15.

A classic study by Dr. Ellen L. Idler Ellen L. Idler (1987). "Religious Involvement and the Health of the Elderly: Some Hypotheses and an Initial Test." *Social Forces* 66: 226–238.

136   *According to Dr. C. R. Snyder* C. R. Synder (2000). "The Past and Possible Futures of Hope." *Journal of Social and Clinical Psychology* 19: 11–28.

"Goals are the targets of mental action sequences" Ibid., p. 13.

"To reach such goals" Ibid.

"A motivational component—agency" Ibid.

137   *greater hope is associated with less depression* T. R. Elliott, T. E. Witty, S. Herrick, and J. T. Hoffman (1991). "Negotiating Reality After Physical Loss: Hope, Depression, and Disability." *Journal of Personality and Social Psychology* 61: 608–613.

avoidance of behaviors that prolong recovery D. D. Barnum, C. R. Synder, M. A. Rapoff, M. M. Mani, and R. Thompson (1998). "Hope and Social Support in the Psychological Adjustment of Pediatric Burn Survivors and Matched Controls." *Children's Health Care* 27: 15–30.

less physical pain in response to stress Synder, op. cit.

greater health-related knowledge L. M. Irving, C. R. Synder, and J. J. Crowson Jr. (1998). "Hope and Coping with Cancer by College Women." *Journal of Personality* 22: 195–214.

Dr. Harold G. Koenig, Duke psychiatrist and researcher Harold G. Koenig (1994). "Religion and Hope for the Disabled Elder." In *Religion in Aging and Health: Theoretical Foundations and Methodological Frontiers*, edited by Jeffrey S. Levin. Newbury Park, Calif.: Sage Publications; pp. 18–51.

religious faith "provides a mechanism" Ibid., p. 30.

"The degree of hope and emotional strength" Ibid.

Dr. Koenig described eleven characteristics of faith   Ibid., pp. 30–31.

138 *religious scholar Dr. John Bowker described how each of the world's major religions*
John Bowker (1970). *Problems of Suffering in Religions of the World.* Cambridge, England:
Cambridge University Press.

Still, precisely because the "realities of suffering are common to us all"   Ibid., p. 4.

Whether one's faith is based upon illusions or upon truth   Jerome D. Frank (1975).
"Mind-Body Relationships in Illness and Healing." *Journal of the International Academy of
Preventive Medicine* 2(3): 46–59.

"expectant faith can be healing"   Ibid., p. 53.

139 **Spontaneous Remission**, *an annotated bibliography*   Brendan O'Regan and Caryle
Hirshberg (1993). *Spontaneous Remission: An Annotated Bibliography.* Sausalito, Calif.: Institute of Noetic Sciences.

These include remission of cancerous tumors   Ibid., pp. 53–348.

Also documented were remission of   Ibid., pp. 349–502.

one of which they termed "faith/positive outcome expectancy"   Ibid., p. 45.

"belief in disease as a direct reflection of mental state"   Marcia Angell (1985). "Disease as
a Reflection of the Psyche." *New England Journal of Medicine* 312: 1570–1572; esp. p. 1572.

140 *"When a patient stands on the firm ground of religious belief"*   Viktor Frankl (1984;
original, 1946). *Man's Search for Meaning*, revised and updated. New York: Washington
Square Press; pp. 141–142.

Dr. Norman Vincent Peale's famous "power of positive thinking"   Norman Vincent
Peale (1996; original, 1952). *The Power of Positive Thinking.* New York: Ballantine Books.

"Does optimism promote health?"   Shelley E. Taylor (1989). *Positive Illusions: Creative
Self-Deception and the Healthy Mind.* New York: Basic Books; p. 108.

141 *"Research concerning the relationship of optimism"*   Ibid., p. 111.

the best explanation "for the beneficial impact of unrealistic optimism"   Ibid., p. 115.

"How does the placebo effect occur?"   Ibid., p. 118.

142 *"There is no direct physical response"*   Andrew Weil (1988). *Health and Healing*, revised
and updated. Boston: Houghton Mifflin; p. 209.

No surprise, then, that placebos have been called "a hidden asset in healing"   Brendan
O'Regan (1985). "Placebo—The Hidden Asset in Healing." *Investigations* (a research bulletin of the Institute of Noetic Sciences) 2(1): 1–3.

"Any person will respond to a placebo"   Ibid., p. 210.

143 *This is defined by epidemiologists as measures that promote health*   Hugh Rodman
Leavell and E. Gurney Clark (1958). "Levels of Application of Preventive Medicine." In
Preventive Medicine for the Doctor in His Community: An Epidemiologic Approach, 2nd ed.,
edited by Hugh Rodman Leavell and E. Gurney Clark. New York: McGraw-Hill;
pp. 20–21.

This is defined by epidemiologists as measures that prevent the spread of disease   Ibid., p. 25.

"By faith, by virtue and energy"   Juan Mascaró (trans.) (1973). *The Dhammapada: The
Path of Perfection.* Harmondsworth, England: Penguin Books.

144 *"Following the way from the start"*   D. C. Lau (trans.) (1963). *Lao Tzu: Tao Te Ching.*
Harmondsworth, England: Penguin Books.

"Allah is all-sufficient"   N. J. Dawood (trans.) (1974). *The Koran.* Harmondsworth, England: Penguin Books.

"Those who ever follow my doctrine"   Juan Mascaró (trans.) (1962). *The Bhagavad Gita.*
Harmondsworth, England: Penguin Books.

145 *Further, the combination of factors*   Levin (2000), op. cit.

146 *"I believe that understanding the mechanisms"*   Ian Wickramasekera (1999). "The Faith
Factor, the Placebo, and AAPB: The Placebo Is a Conditioned Response Composed of
Credible Expectation and Vivid Memories of Health and Past Healing Events." *AAPB
News and Events* (Spring): 1A–3A.

147 *In their book* **Remarkable Recovery**   Caryle Hirshberg and Marc Ian Barasch (1995).
     *Remarkable Recovery: What Extraordinary Healings Tell Us About Getting Well and Staying
     Well.* New York: Riverhead Books.

148 *hope and optimism "were of significant benefit"*   Ibid., p. 307.
     what epidemiologists term "coherent"   Judith S. Mausner and Shira Kramer (1985).
     Mausner and Bahn Epidemiology: An Introductory Text, 2nd ed. Philadelphia: W.B. Saunders
     Company; p. 186.

156 *relevant health indicators. These can include*   Jeffrey S. Levin, Thomas A. Glass,
     Lawrence H. Kushi, John R. Schuck, Lea Steele, and Wayne B. Jonas (1997). "Quantita-
     tive Methods in Research on Complementary and Alternative Medicine: A Methodologi-
     cal Manifesto." *Medical Care* 35: 1079–1094.

157 *Using nationally representative data on 1,481 adults*   Jeffrey S. Levin (1993). "Age Dif-
     ferences in Mystical Experiences." *The Gerontologist* 33: 507–513.
     In comparison with data collected in the 1970s   Andrew M. Greeley (1975). *The Sociology
     of the Paranormal: A Reconnaissance.* Beverly Hills, Calif.: Sage Publications.
     the nirvana of Buddhist and Jaina mystics   Heinrich Zimmer (1951). *Philosophies of India.*
     Bollingen Series, no. 26. Princeton, N.J.: Princeton University Press; p. 183.

158 *as in the so-called Toronto blessing*   Margaret M. Poloma and Lynette F. Hoelter (1998).
     "The 'Toronto Blessing': A Holistic Model of Healing." *Journal for the Scientific Study of Re-
     ligion* 37: 257–272.
     hypnagogic or hypnopompic states between wakefulness and sleep   Andreas Mavromatis
     (1987). *Hypnagogia: The Unique State of Consciousness Between Wakefulness and Sleep.* London:
     Routledge.
     attained by shamans and healers   Ralph G. Locke and Edward F. Kelly (1985). "A Pre-
     liminary Model for the Cross-Cultural Analysis of Altered States of Consciousness." *Ethos*
     13: 3–55.
     what they termed "diabolical experiences"   Nicholas P. Spanos and Patricia Moretti
     (1988). "Correlates of Mystical and Diabolical Experiences in a Sample of Female Univer-
     sity Students." *Journal for the Scientific Study of Religion* 27: 105–116.

159 *One study examined the separate effects*   J. E. Kennedy, H. Kanthamani, and John
     Palmer (1994). "Psychic and Spiritual Experiences, Health, Well-Being, and Meaning in
     Life." *Journal of Parapsychology* 58: 353–383.

160 *In a subsequent study, Dr. Kennedy examined*   J. E. Kennedy and H. Kanthamani
     (1995). "An Exploratory Study of the Effects of Paranormal and Spiritual Experience on
     People's Lives and Well-Being." *Journal of the American Society for Psychical Research* 89:
     249–264.

161 *One very interesting study*   Bernard Spilka, George A. Brown, and Stephen A. Cassidy
     (1992). "The Structure of Religious Mystical Experience in Relation to Pre- and Postex-
     perience Lifestyles." *International Journal for the Psychology of Religion* 2: 241–257.

162 *"In the area of epidemiology, the influence of extrasensory factors"*   Louise Mead
     Riscalla (1976). "The Influence of Extrasensory Factors upon Health." *Social Science and
     Medicine* 10: 315–316; esp. p. 315.
     the complex "web of causation"   Brian MacMahon, T. F. Pugh, and J. Ipsen (1960). *Epi-
     demiologic Methods.* Boston: Little, Brown and Company; p. 18.

163 *"A pantheistic…force"*   Jeffrey S. Levin and Harold Y. Vanderpool (1989), op. cit., p. 75.

164 *"This term implies no judgment"*   Jeffrey S. Levin (1996). "How Prayer Heals: A Theo-
     retical Model." *Alternative Therapies in Health and Medicine* 2 (1): 66–73; p. 69.

165 *Harvard physician Dr. Herbert Benson described physiological changes*   Herbert Benson
     (1975). *The Relaxation Response.* New York: Avon Books.
     These techniques bring on "bodily changes"   Ibid., p. 26.
     these methods of self-regulation have "always existed"   Ibid.

contemplative prayers of Christian monastics Jacob Needleman (1980). *Lost Christianity: A Journey of Rediscovery to the Center of Christian Experience*. Toronto: Bantam New Age.

meditative practices of Jewish Kabbalists Aryeh Kaplan (1995; original, 1978). *Meditation and the Bible*. Northvale, N.J.: Jason Aronson.

Sufi mystics Idries Shah (1974). *The Way of the Sufi*. London: Penguin Books.

Dr. Benson compared a variety of religious and secular practices Benson, op. cit., pp. 98–99.

although scientists continue to debate the evidence David S. Holmes (1984). "Meditation and Somatic Arousal Reduction: A Review of the Experimental Evidence." *American Psychologist* 39: 1–10.

"increase in intensity and frequency" Benson, op. cit., p. 90.

They are linked to Michael Hutchison (1991). *Mega Brain New Tools and Techniques for Brain Growth and Mind Expansion*, revised and updated. New York: Ballantine Books.

166 *A team of anthropologists from Los Angeles* Dureen J. Hughes and Norbert T. Melville (1990). "Changes in Brainwave Activity during Trance Channeling: A Pilot Study." *Journal of Transpersonal Psychology* 22: 175–189.

This activity is "performed in an altered state" Ibid., p. 176.

It was concluded that there are "definite neurophysiological correlates" Ibid., p. 184.

167 *A provocative study by scientists at the University of Louisville* Walter W. Surwillo and Doug-las P. Hobson (1978). "Brain Electrical Activity During Prayer." *Psychological Reports* 43: 135–143.

According to investigators, "There is no evidence of EEG slowing" Ibid., p. 139.

often "show an acceleration in frequency" Ibid., p. 142.

168 *I investigated the association between "intrinsic" and "extrinsic" religiousness* Jeffrey S. Levin, Ian E. Wickramasekera, and Caryle Hirshberg (1998). "Is Religiousness a Correlate of Absorption?: Implications for Psychophysiology, Coping, and Morbidity." *Alternative Therapies in Health and Medicine* 4(6): 72–76.

"self-altering experiences" Suzanne M. Roche and Kevin M. McConkey (1990). "Absorption: Nature, Assessment, and Correlates." *Journal of Personality and Social Psychology* 59: 91–101.

They derive, respectively, from psychologist Dr. Gordon Allport's concepts Gordon W. Allport (1954). *The Nature of Prejudice*. Reading, Mass.: Addison-Wesley.

169 *including the Religious Orientation Scale (ROS)* Gordon W. Allport and J. Michael Ross (1967). "Personal Religious Orientation and Prejudice." *Journal of Personality and Social Psychology* 5: 432–443.

Our sample comprised 83 adults in a pilot study Caryle Hirshberg and Marc Ian Barasch (1995). *Remarkable Recovery: What Extraordinary Healings Tell Us About Getting Well and Staying Well*. New York: Riverhead Books; pp. 324–334.

170 *in the Greens' book* **Beyond Biofeedback** Elmer Green and Alyce Green (1977). *Beyond Biofeedback*. Fort Wayne, Ind.: Knoll Publishing Company.

"It is most amazing that people do not understand" Ibid., p. 207.

171 *In Book Three of the* **Yoga Sutras** James Haughton Woods (trans.) (1914). *The Yoga-System of Patañjali of the Ancient Hindu Doctrine of Concentration of Mind Embracing the Mnemonic Rules, Called Yoga-Sutras, of Patañjali and the Comment, Called Yoga-Bhashya, Attributed to Veda Vyasa and the Explanation, Called Tattva-Vaiçcaradi, of Vachaspati-Miçra*. Delhi, India: Motilal Banarsidass.

a book called **Science Studies Yoga** James Funderburk (1977). *Science Studies Yoga: A Review of Physiological Data*. Honesdale, Penn.: Himalayan International Institute of Yoga Science and Philosophy.

172 *Over the years, I have found upwards of fifty to sixty names* Levin and Vanderpool, op. cit., p. 75.

Mary Coddington (1990). *Seekers of the Healing Energy: Reich, Cayce, the Kahunas, and Other Masters of the Vital Force.* Rochester, Vt.: Healing Arts Press.

Robert Anton Wilson (1987). *Wilhelm Reich in Hell.* Phoenix, Ariz.: Falcon Press.

L. F. Ludzia (1987). *Life Force: The Secret of Empowerment.* St. Paul, Minn.: Llewellyn Publications.

William Collinge (1998). *Subtle Energy: Awakening to the Unseen Forces in Our Lives.* New York: Warner Books.

173   *Respected scientists debate the interrelationships*   Jeff Levin (1998). "A Message from the President." *Bridges: Magazine of the International Society for the Study of Subtle Energies and Energy Medicine* 9 (1): 3, 14.

sophisticated models of "psychoenergetic systems"   A. J. Ruttenbur (1979). "Introduction to the General System Basis of Psychoenergetics." In *Psychoenergetic Systems: The Interaction of Consciousness, Energy and Matter,* edited by Stanley Krippner. New York: Gordon and Breach Science Publishers; pp. xvii–xxvi.

the "human bioenergetic system"   Richard Gerber (1988). *Vibrational Medicine: New Choices for Healing Ourselves.* Santa Fe, N.M: Bear and Company; p. 420.

"extrapersonal" and "transpersonal" states of consciousness   Elmer E. Green and Alyce M. Green (1986). "Biofeedback and States of Consciousness." In *Handbook of States of Consciousness,* edited by Benjamin B. Wolman and Montague Ullman. New York: Van Nostrand Reinhold; pp. 553–589.

Dr. William Collinge, in his book   William Collinge (1998). "Courting the Spirit: Subtle Energies in Prayer, Meditation, and Healing." *Subtle Energy: Awakening to the Unseen Forces in Our Lives.* New York: Warner Books; pp. 225–271.

176   *The noted sociologist of religion Dr. Andrew M. Greeley*   Andrew M. Greeley (1987). "Hallucinations among the Widowed." *Social Science Research* 71: 258–265.

"a clearly religious belief structure"   Nils G. Holm (1982). "Mysticism and Intense Experience." *Journal for the Scientific Study of Religion* 21: 268–276; esp. p. 275.

177   *members of parapsychological research societies*   Leanne M. Williams and Harvey J. Irwin (1991). "A Study of Paranormal Belief, Magical Ideation as an Index of Schizotypy and Cognitive Style." *Personality and Individual Differences* 12: 1339–1348.

may "represent a cognitive 'defense'"   Ibid., p. 1339.

A study at Louisiana Tech University   Jerome Tobacyk and Gary Milford (1983). "Belief in Paranormal Phenomena: Assessment Instrument Development and Implications for Personality Functioning." *Journal of Personality and Social Psychology* 44: 1029–1037.

"Self-actualization is a lifestyle"   Joseph B. Tamney (1992). "Religion and Self-Actualization." In *Religion and Mental Health,* edited by John F. Schumaker. New York: Oxford University Press; p. 136.

178   *According to philosopher Dr. Mark B. Woodhouse*   Mark B. Woodhouse (1996). *Paradigm Wars: Worldviews for a New Age.* Berkeley, Calif.: Frog, Ltd.; pp. 205–249.

identified "a generic core in mystical experiences"   Ibid., p. 216.

"No serious student of mysticism would argue"   Ibid.

184   *established Western religions such as Roman Catholicism*   Francis MacNutt (1974). *Healing.* Toronto: Bantam Books.

mainline Protestantism   Agnes Sanford (1972). *The Healing Light,* rev. ed. New York: Ballantine Books.

evangelical Christianity   Roger F. Hurding (1986). "Healing." In *Medicine and the Bible,* edited by Bernard Palmer. Exeter, England: The Paternoster Press; pp. 191–216.

Judaism   Julius Preuss (1993; original, 1911). *Biblical and Talmudic Medicine.* Translated and edited by Fred Rosner. Northvale, N.J.: Jason Aronson Inc.; p. 27.

Alice Bailey's Lucis Trust   Alice A. Bailey (1953). *Esoteric Healing.* vol. 4 of *A Treatise on the Seven Rays.* New York: Lucis Publishing Company.

the Theosophical Society   H. Tudor Edmunds and Associates (1976; original, 1944). *Some Unrecognized Factors in Medicine*. Wheaton, Ill.: The Theosophical Publishing House.

Theosophical Research Centre (1968). *The Mystery of Healing*, revised edition. Wheaton, Ill.: The Theosophical Publishing House.

Rudolf Steiner's Anthroposophical Society   Rudolf Steiner (1981; original, 1961). *Health & Illness*, vol. 1: *Nine Lectures to the Workmen at the Goetheanum, Dornach, Switzerland*. Translated by Maria St. Goar. Spring Valley, N.Y.: The Anthroposophic Press.

Max Freedom Long's Huna Research Associates   Max Freedom Long (1953). *The Secret Science at Work*. Marina del Rey, Calif.: DeVorss & Company.

Manly P. Hall's Philosophical Research Society   Manly P. Hall (1972; original, 1944). *Healing: The Divine Art*. Los Angeles: Philosophical Research Society.

is a "means of access to the cosmic consciousness"   Pierre Marinier (1954). "Reflections on Prayer: Its Causes and Its Psychophysiological Effects." In *Forms and Techniques of Altruistic and Spiritual Growth*, edited by Pitirim A. Sorokin. Boston: Beacon Press; p. 158.

185   *The most famous study of absent prayer*   Randolph C. Byrd (1988). "Positive Therapeutic Effects of Intercessory Prayer in a Coronary Care Unit Population." *Southern Medical Journal* 81: 826–829.

"suggest that intercessory prayer to the Judeo-Christian God"   Ibid., p. 826.

186   *Quite the contrary, reasoned a follow-up correspondent*   G. A. Reich (1989). "Religion and Medicine." Letter to the editor in *Southern Medical Journal* 82: 670.

notably the four-volume **Healing Research**   Daniel J. Benor (1992). *Healing Research: Holistic Energy Medicine and Spirituality*, vol. 1: *Research in Healing*. Munich, Germany: Helix.

According to Dr. Jerry Solfvin   Jerry Solfvin (1984). "Mental Healing." In *Advances in Parapsychological Research*, vol. 4, edited by Stanley Krippner. Jefferson, N.C.: McFarland and Company; pp. 31–63.

"A wide variety of specific practices and techniques"   Ibid., p. 31.

187   *Still, according to Dr. Larry Dossey*   Larry Dossey (1998). "Prayer, Medicine, and Science: The New Dialogue." In *Scientific and Pastoral Perspectives on Intercessory Prayer: An Exchange Between Larry Dossey, M.D., and Health Care Chaplains*, edited by Larry VandeCreek. New York: The Haworth Pastoral Press; pp. 7–37.

"Part of the problem in identifying work"   Ibid., pp. 10–11.

A California researcher conducted   Daniel P. Wirth (1990). "The Effect of Noncontact Therapeutic Touch (NCTT) on the Healing Rate of Full Thickness Dermal Wounds." *Subtle Energies* 1: 1–20.

188   *California researchers investigated*   R. N. Miller (1982). "Study on the Effectiveness of Remote Mental Healing." *Medical Hypotheses* 8: 481–490.

half were randomly assigned to a control group   Benor, op. cit., pp. 215–216.

a four-step prayer called Spiritual Mind Treatment   Miller, op. cit., p. 481.

189   *a team of medical scientists from University Hospital in Utrecht*   Jaap J. Beutler, Johannes T. M. Attevelt, Sybo A. Schouten, Joop A. J. Faber, Evert J. Dorhout Mees, and Gijsbert G. Geijskes (1988). "Paranormal Healing and Hypertension." *British Medical Journal* 296: 1491–1494.

A researcher at the University of Connecticut Health Center   Bruce Greyson (1996). "Distance Healing of Patients with Major Depression." *Journal of Scientific Exploration* 10: 447–465.

190   *This involved seeking "to induce through meditation"*   Ibid., p. 453.

The investigator concluded that "the distance healing did exert"   Ibid., p. 462.

A study recently published in the **Western Journal of Medicine**   Fred Sicher, Elisabeth Targ, Dan Moore II, and Helene S. Smith (1998). "A Randomized Double-Blind Study of the Effect of Distant Healing in a Population with Advanced AIDS: Report of a Small Scale Study." *Western Journal of Medicine* 169: 356–363.

191   *"Practically anyone's prayers appeared effective"*   Larry Dossey (1997). "Running Scared: How We Hide from Who We Are." *Alternative Therapies in Health and Medicine* 3 (2): 8–15; p. 8.

he noted, "At this time, research on prayer"   Michael E. McCullough (1995). "Prayer and Health: Conceptual Issues, Research Review, and Research Agenda." *Journal of Psychology and Theology* 23: 15–29; esp. p. 20.

192   *In an interesting article*   Paul N. Duckro and Philip R. Magaletta (1994). "The Effect of Prayer on Physical Health: Experimental Evidence." *Journal of Religion and Health* 33: 211–219.

"Demonstrating positive outcomes"   Ibid., pp. 217–218.

In 1997, I was solicited by JAMA   Jeffrey S. Levin, David B. Larson, and Christina M. Puchalski (1997), op. cit.

193   *The series, called "Religious Healing"*   Alice E. Paulsen (1926). "Religious Healing: Preliminary Report." *Journal of the American Medical Association* 86: 1519–1522, 1617–1623, 1692–1697.

"It may well be that religious healing"   Ibid., p. 1694.

194   *"The medical profession has largely ignored"*   Ibid., p. 1696.

In 1997, I published my own take   Jeffrey S. Levin (1996). "How Prayer Heals: A Theoretical Model." *Alternative Therapies in Health and Medicine* 2: 66–73.

195   *According to physicists*   Fred Alan Wolf (1981). *Taking the Quantum Leap: The New Physics for Nonscientists.* San Francisco, Calif.: Harper and Row.

"the statistical predictions of quantum"   Levin, op. cit., p. 69.

The concept of nonlocality was first fleshed out   David Bohm (1980). *Wholeness and the Implicate Order.* London: Ark.

"At the level of our everyday lives"   Michael Talbot (1991). *The Holographic Universe.* New York: HarperPerennial; p. 41.

nonlocality is not just a concept debated by scientists   John P. Briggs and F. David Peat (1984). *Looking Glass Universe: The Emerging Science of Wholeness.* New York: Cornerstone Library.

196   *This amounts to asserting "that there is no here and there"*   Ibid., p. 89.

"then we live in a nonlocal universe"   Gary Zukav (1979). *The Dancing Wu Li Masters: An Overview of the New Physics.* Toronto: Bantam Books; p. 302.

suffers acutely from what he termed "physics envy"   Larry Dossey (1984). *Beyond Illness: Discovering the Experience of Health.* Boston: Shambhala; p. 16.

"Dossey describes this as a reliance"   Jeffrey S. Levin (1988). Book review of *Beyond Illness: Discovering the Experience of Health* by Larry Dossey, in *Journal of Religion and Health* 27: 329–330.

he introduced the concept of "nonlocal mind"   Larry Dossey (1989). *Recovering the Soul: A Scientific and Spiritual Search.* New York: Bantam Books; pp. 178–186.

"If the mind is nonlocal in space and time"   Ibid., p. 7.

197   *"The confirmation of this principle of nonlocality"*   Jeffrey Mishlove (1993). *The Roots of Consciousness: The Classic Encyclopedia of Consciousness Studies*, revised and expanded. Tulsa, Okla.: Council Oaks Books; p. 316.

198   *I proposed naturalistic explanations*   Jeffrey S. Levin (1993). "Esoteric vs. Exoteric Explanations for Findings Linking Spirituality and Health." *Advances: The Journal of Mind-Body Health* 9 (4): 54–56.

"For example, experiencing the presence of a healer"   Ibid., p. 55.

terms such as "paraphysical" or "magnetic"   David Aldridge (1993). "Is There Evidence for Spiritual Healing?" *Advances: The Journal of Mind-Body Health* 9 (4): 4–21.

"extended mind"   Rupert L. Sheldrake (1994). "Prayer: A Challenge for Science." *Noetic Sciences Review* 30: 5–9.

"morphic fields" Rupert Sheldrake (1988). *The Presence of the Past: Morphic Resonance and the Habits of Nature*. New York: Vintage Books.

"nonlocal mind" Larry Dossey (1994). "Healing and the Mind: Is There a Dark Side?" *Journal of Scientific Exploration* 8: 73–90.

"transpersonal" Ibid.

"psi" Charles T. Tart (1986). *Waking Up: Overcoming the Obstacles to Human Potential*. Boston: New Science Library.

"consciousness" Stanley Krippner and Alberto Villodo (1986). *The Realms of Healing*, 3rd ed. Berkeley, Calif.: Celestial Arts.

199 *The fact that these phenomena may seem to "violate the tenets"* Levin (1996), op. cit., p. 69.

"While not a universal conception of the deity" Jeffrey S. Levin (in press). "The Spiritual Basis of Health and Healing." In *Textbook of Complementary and Alternative Medicine*, edited by Wayne B. Jonas, Jeffrey S. Levin, and George T. Lewith. Philadelphia: Lippincott Williams and Wilkins.

200 *"The idea that there is such a Being"* Ibid.

Dr. Byrd stated, "I thank God for responding" Byrd, op. cit., p. 829.

201 *we can safely say that religion and health are connected* Jeffrey S. Levin (1994). "Religion and Health: Is There an Association, Is It Valid, and Is It Causal?" *Social Science and Medicine* 38: 1475–1482.

202 *Dr. Larry Dossey has collected some of the more hilarious* Dossey (1998), op. cit., p. 22.

"This is the kind of thing that I would not believe" Editorial (1976). "Scanning the Issue." *Proceedings of the IEEE* 64 (3): 291. Cited in *Mind-Reach: Scientists Look at Psychic Ability*, by Russell Targ and Harold Puthoff (1977). New York: Delta; p. 169.

206 *modern scientific medicine has passed through two eras* Dossey (1989), op. cit., pp. 263–267.

will come to accept evidence that "minds are spread" Ibid., p. 265.

207 *I have termed this new perspective* Jeff Levin (2000). "From Psychosomatic to Theosomatic: The Role of Spirit in the Next New Paradigm." *Subtle Energies and Energy Medicine* 9(1): 1–26.

"Western biomedicine . . . is still wrestling" Jeffrey S. Levin and Harold Y. Vanderpool (1987), op. cit., pp. 590–591.

208 *"To omit the spiritual element"* Larry Dossey (1995). "Whatever Happened to Healers?" *Alternative Therapies in Health and Medicine* 1 (5): 6–13; esp. p. 12.

210 *and "complete surrender to the will"* Ibid., p. 301.

211 *In his classic **Dynamics of Faith*** Paul Tillich (1957). *Dynamics of Faith*. New York: Harper Colophon Books.

faith can be defined as "ultimate concern" Ibid., p. 1.

It may be "the Mosaic law" Ibid., p. 88.

we can tap into something "unconditional" Ibid., p. 8.

Tillich asserted, "It precedes" Ibid., p. 110.

*described in works such as **The Secret Doctrine*** H. P. Blavatsky (1970; original, 1888). *The Secret Doctrine: The Synthesis of Science, Religion, and Philosophy*. Pasadena, Calif.: Theosophical University Press.

212 *the "primordial tradition"* Luc Benoist (1988; original, 1963). *The Esoteric Path: An Introduction to the Hermetic Tradition*. Wellingborough, England: Crucible; p. 29.

"secret wisdom" David Conway (1985). *Secret Wisdom: The Occult Universe Explored*. London: Jonathan Cape.

"forgotten truth" Huston Smith (1976). *Forgotten Truth: The Primordial Tradition*. New York: Harper and Row.

"ancient theology" Joscelyn Godwin (1979). *Athanasius Kircher: A Renaissance Man and the Quest for Lost Knowledge*. London: Thames and Hudson; p. 18.

"ageless wisdom"   Bailey, op. cit., p. 2.

each represents the manifestation of a human being   I. K. Taimni (1969). *Man, God and the Universe.* Wheaton, Ill.: Quest.

Some healers and intuitives claim to be able   A. E. Powell (1983; original, 1925). *The Etheric Double: The Health Aura of Man.* Wheaton, Ill.: Theosophical Publishing House, pp. 74–78.

The building blocks of this dimension   A. E. Powell (1982; original, 1927). *The Astral Body and Other Astral Phenomena.* Wheaton, Ill.: Theosophical Publishing House; pp. 4–10.
     Arthur E. Powell (1967; original 1927). *The Mental Body.* London: Theosophical Publishing House; pp. 7–12.

213   *"the receptacle of all that is enduring"*   Arthur E. Powell (1972; original, 1928). *The Causal Body and the Ego.* London: Theosophical Publishing House; p. 90.

In the Native American medical tradition   Ken "Bear Hawk" Cohen (1999). "Native American Medicine." In *Essentials of Complementary and Alternative Medicine,* edited by Wayne B. Jonas and Jeffrey S. Levin. Philadelphia: Lippincott Williams and Wilkins; pp. 233–251.

"Health and disease," Cohen has noted   Ibid., p. 236.

all things are connected and "part of a single whole"   Ibid.

214   *has called "Hebraic medicine"*   Gerald Epstein (1987). "Hebraic Medicine." *Advances: The Journal of Mind-Body Health* 4 (1): 56–66.

produced Ayurvedic medicine   Vasant Lad (1984). *Ayurveda: The Science of Self-Healing.* Santa Fe, N.M.: Lotus Press.

came Tibetan medicine   Sogyal Rinpoche (1999). "The Spiritual Heart of Tibetan Medicine: Its Contribution to the Modern World." *Alternative Therapies in Health and Medicine* 5 (3): 70–72.

traditional Chinese medicine grew   Lixing Lao (1999). "Traditional Chinese Medicine." In *Essentials of Complementary and Alternative Medicine,* edited by Wayne B. Jonas and Jeffrey S. Levin. Philadelphia: Lippincott Williams and Wilkins; pp. 216–232.

the Unani medical system has flourished   Helen Sheehan and S. J. Hussain (in press). "Unani Tibb." In *Textbook of Complementary and Alternative Medicine,* edited by Wayne B. Jonas, Jeffrey S. Levin, and George T. Lewith. Philadelphia: Lippincott Williams and Wilkins.

notably Anthroposophical medicine   Michael Evans and Iain Rodger (1992). *Anthroposophical Medicine: Healing for Body, Soul and Spirit.* London: Thorsons.

the teachings of Edgar Cayce   Reba Ann Karp (1986). *Edgar Cayce Encyclopedia of Healing.* New York: Warner Books.

Dr. Epstein identified and described a "Western spiritual medical tradition"   Heidi E. Rain (1993). "The Western Spiritual Medical Tradition: An Interview with Gerald Epstein, M.D." *Body Mind Spirit* (November/December): 39–43.

One encyclopedic compendium of medical knowledge   Julius Preuss (1993; original, 1911). *Biblical and Talmudic Medicine.* Translated and edited by Fred Rosner. Northvale, N.J.: Jason Aronson Inc.

the "bodymind unity"   Epstein, op. cit., p. 60.

215   *This in turn "requires a degree of faith"*   Ibid.

by "[r]emembering God"   Rain, op. cit., p. 43.

Despite research evidence   Jeffrey S. Levin (1994). "Investigating the Epidemiologic Effects of Religious Experience: Findings, Explanations, and Barriers." In *Religion in Aging and Health: Theoretical Foundations and Methodological Frontier,* edited by Jeffrey S. Levin. Thousand Oaks, Calif.: Sage Publications; pp. 3–17.

Physicians rarely inquire about the spiritual life of their patients   Harold G. Koenig, George R. Parkerson Jr., and Keith G. Meador (1997). "Religion Index for Psychiatric Research." Letter to the editor, in *American Journal of Psychiatry* 153: 885–886.

a category describing disruptions in one's religious or spiritual life Robert P. Turner, David Lukoff, Ruth Tiffany Barnhouse, and Francis G. Lu (1995). "Religious or Spiritual Problem: A Culturally Sensitive Diagnostic Category in the DSM-IV." *Journal of Nervous and Mental Disease* 183: 435–444.

216 *including mystical and near-death experiences* Ibid., pp. 439–440.

"In the face of psychiatry's long-standing tendency" Ibid., pp. 442–443.

At the same time, medical educators have begun Christina M. Puchalski and David B. Larson (1998). "Developing Curricula in Spirituality and Medicine." *Academic Medicine* 73: 970–974.

217 *About a hundred medical schools have applied* Ibid., pp. 972–973.

In a review published in Academic Medicine Ibid., p. 973.

218 *The Templeton Foundation published* David B. Larson, James P. Swyers, and Michael E. McCullough (eds.) (1998). *Scientific Research on Spirituality and Health.* (A report based on the Scientific Progress in Spirituality Conferences.) Rockville, Md.: National Institute for Healthcare Research.

The National Institute for Healthcare Research published David B. Larson and Susan S. Larson (1994). *The Forgotten Factor in Physical and Mental Health: What Does the Research Show?—An Independent Study Seminar.* Rockville, Md.: National Institute for Healthcare Research.

A recent Fetzer Institute publication Fetzer Institute/National Institute on Aging (1999). *Multidimensional Measurement of Religiousness/Spirituality for Use in Health Research.* Kalamazoo, Mich.: John E. Fetzer Institute.

He has especially focused on the role of religion Harold G. Koenig, Harvey J. Cohen, Dan G. Blazer, Carl Pieper, Keith G. Meador, Frank Shelp, Veeraindar Goli, and Bob DiPasquale (1992). "Religious Coping and Depression Among Elderly, Hospitalized Medically Ill Men." *American Journal of Psychiatry* 149: 1693–1700.

219 *This theme is taken up in Dr. Koenig's book* Harold G. Koenig (1999). *The Healing Power of Faith: Science Explores Medicine's Last Great Frontier.* New York: Simon and Schuster.

Articulated in the 1970s by Dr. George L. Engel George L. Engel (1977). "The Need for a New Medical Model: A Challenge for Biomedicine." *Science* 196: 129–136.

220 *I believe that as the new theosomatic medical model* Jeff Levin (1998). "A Message from the President." *Bridges: Magazine of the International Society for the Study of Subtle Energies and Energy Medicine* 9 (2): 8–9.

In 1995, Dr. Richard L. Garrison Richard L. Garrison (1995). "The Five Generations of American Medical Revolutions." *Journal of Family Practice* 40: 281–287.

221 *"Many authors say that we are surrounded"* Ibid., p. 281.

222 *"The time for attempting to repair"* Ibid., p. 286.

a "spectrum of consciousness" Ken Wilber (1977). *The Spectrum of Consciousness.* Wheaton, Ill.: Quest.

Index

About the Author

Jeff Levin, Ph.D., M.P.H., is a social epidemiologist and writer living in Kansas. He was trained in religion, sociology, public health, preventive medicine, and gerontology at Duke University, the University of North Carolina, the University of Texas Medical Branch, and the University of Michigan. From 1989 to 1997, he served on the faculty of the Department of Family and Community Medicine at Eastern Virginia Medical School in Norfolk, Virginia.

Dr. Levin pioneered basic research on the epidemiology of religion. His work has been funded by the U.S. National Institutes of Health, as well as by private sources, including the American Medical Association and the Institute of Noetic Sciences.

Dr. Levin is a senior research fellow of the National Institute for Healthcare Research; an advisory board member of the Center on Aging, Religion, and Spirituality; a board of trustees member of the Shepherd's Centers of America; and a past president of the International Society for the Study of Subtle Energies and Energy Medicine. He has been chairman of the NIH Working Group on Quantitative Methods in Alternative Medicine, is a former member of the NIH Workgroup on Measures of Religiousness and Spirituality, and is a current editorial board member of several peer-reviewed scientific and medical journals.

Dr. Levin is the author of more than 110 scholarly publications, and he has given nearly a hundred conference presentations and invited lectures on the relationship between religion and health. His research has been featured in cover stories in *Time* and *Reader's Digest*, and on National Public Radio.

CPSIA information can be obtained
at www.ICGtesting.com
Printed in the USA
LVHW032200040223
738699LV00006B/31

9 780471 218937